BIPOLAR…..ME?
John Barrett

Copyright © 2012 John Barrett

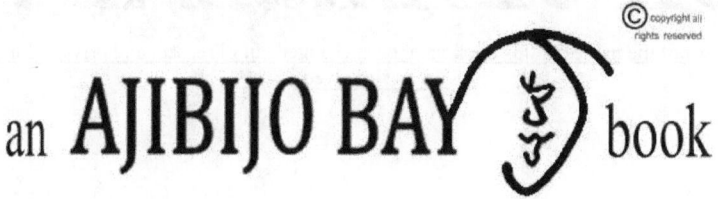

All rights reserved. No part of this publication may be reproduced, stored in a retrieval system, or transmitted in any form or by any means without the prior written permission of the publisher.

I've written this book the way I speak (London accent) or as I hear other people speak, in order for the reader to better understand each character.

BIPOLAR......ME?

Most of the names in this book have been changed out of respect and privacy for those involved

For Lucy

Everything is a state of mind.

Also by the same author

**Frank Fireball in
Pronounced Dop-el-geng-er**

The Adventures of Dustman Dan

Bipolar…..Maybe?
(Volume One)

Bipolar…..Definitely!

**Frank Fireball
and the
Confounding Case
of
Paxomus Maxomus**

A Saturday in Mid September

Writing under the name
Sydney Novak

**An Empty Kettle
(Part 1 and 2)**

With thanks to:

Pauline and Dave, Lee and Sam, Mick and Pauline, my brother Davey, my sister Ellie, my mum and dad and to all the staff, doctors and nurses at the hospital (sorry I was such a pain in the arse)

SECTION 1: HIGH
Page 5 - page 100

SECTION 2: MEDIUM
Page 101 - page 259

SECTION 3: LOW
Page 260 - page 369

SECTION 4: GETTING BETTER
Page 370 - page 395

SECTION 5: BETTER?
Page 396 - page 406

SECTION 1: HIGH

CHAPTER 1

19th September 2008, somewhere in Essex….

After twenty years and one day short of one month, I split up with my wife. Things hadn't been going well for the last couple of years and I had left for about a month, the year before. We both decided to try and work it out but after moving back in, it was clear that things hadn't improved. I suppose owing to the fact we had been together for so long (I met her when I was nineteen) it just seemed wrong to be separated. Like so many couples, we had fallen out of love and when that happens, there is no point living together. I just felt it was best that the kids didn't see us arguing all the time and I'm sure she agreed. I moved to a small village about nine miles away, into a one bedroom flat and was working as a self-employed builder. The economic situation was starting to get decidedly dodgy and I was earning my income on a day to day basis. We had always struggled to make a decent living and when the family business went into liquidation during the previous recession back in the mid-nineties, my wife saw an advert in the newsagent's window for an ironing service which paid so much per bag of washing. She quickly realised that she could earn more money starting up her own business and the work load steadily increased. I had always felt that she was such a hard worker and have total respect for my wife but after I left and over the next few months, I had unfounded ill feelings towards

SECTION 1: HIGH

her. My family's business was in packaging and when I left school as soon as I turned sixteen, I started working there and along with my cousin Mick, who is eighteen years older than me, I became a director of the firm at the age of twenty one. This may sound great and it was for about the first two and a half years but when things started to get tough, it became a nightmare. It was the time of the recession in the nineties and small businesses were folding left right and centre. When you have a family run company which has been going since before World War Two, you try everything possible to keep it going because you somehow feel responsible to all the people who had worked there previously. We borrowed money off other family members and friends but it was all to no avail. Looking back now, I realise that I was still a kid and didn't have much life experience and all the hardships you face can actually help put your life on a better course. Luckily I had a friend who also ran a family business, manufacturing wooden pasting tables and step ladders and he offered me the post of production manager which I snapped up. Although I will always be grateful to him, it was so hard working for someone else when you had been your own boss. I worked for my friend's family for nine years and during all of that time, I wanted to be my own boss again but my self confidence had taken a bit of a nose dive. His company was also falling on hard times and I felt that anything to do with manufacturing in this country was rapidly drying up. My father-in-law was a property developer and me and my wife suggested that I go in with him, which he agreed to but warned us that times were getting tougher and it wasn't as easy to sell houses any more and make a good profit. He turned out to be 100% accurate and it seemed that everything I was involved with ended up falling apart. I picked up a few skills in the building trade and decided the best thing to do was work for myself, fitting kitchens, decking etc. This too has its problems (ask anyone in the self-employed building trade) but I just didn't know what else I could do. I had no qualifications whatsoever and at the age of forty one, felt over the hill.

So I moved into my one bedroom flat and the job I was currently working on involved painting over old kitchen units and tiling the floor and walls. It was turning out to be a real pig of a job and the owners were starting to get pissed off at the length of time it was taking. I had so many other things going through my head at the time that my mind just wasn't on the job. It was a Tuesday morning and I was on the dual carriageway at Walthamstow, driving to a builder's merchants to pick up some gear for this particular kitchen job. I must have been doing about sixty when I had a blow out and looking in my rear-view mirror; saw the tyre fly into the air. Luckily, I managed to keep the car under control and pulled over to the side. There wasn't any lay-by and so I had to park on the inside lane with cars and lorries rushing by. I opened up the boot and had to remove most of my tools slung in the back, just so I could get to the jack. The spare tyre was underneath the car, so after loosening the bolts and jacking up the car, I removed the wheel and crawled under to unscrew the spare. As forty foot articulated lorries zoomed past, the car was shaking and I thought I was going to get crushed! Just at that

SECTION 1: HIGH

moment, my mobile rang and it was the lady of the house I was doing the kitchen job for.

"Where are you John, you should have been here fifteen minutes ago!" she said in an angry tone.

"I've had a blow out on the north circular and I'm changing the tyre as we speak"

I could tell that she didn't believe me but by that point, I didn't give a fuck because I kept thinking about my eldest son. At the time, he was at college and I'd asked him if he could take the day off to help me but he said he couldn't. He'd taken a few days off the week before and I suppose I had started to take his help for granted and so when he said he couldn't help on this occasion, I got angry with him. Sorry mate that was obviously part of the bipolar which I knew nothing about at the time. I finally got the wheel changed, threw the jack, spare and tools back in the car, nearly got mowed down trying to get back in again, drove to the builder's merchants, picked up the gear and as I'm getting back in the car, the mobile rings again.

"WHERE ARE YOU?"

"I'LL BE WITH YOU IN TEN FUCKING MINUTES!"

Not good.

I hung up the phone and drove like a maniac to the job, trying to remember if I'd done the wheel nuts up properly. When I arrived, the woman was waiting outside and did not look happy at all.

"How dare you swear at me!" she yelled.

"I wasn't swearing at you, I………." and then I burst out crying which was something I hardly ever did. Again, not good and totally unprofessional. She called her husband to come out, "Tony, you deal with this. I've had enough of him!"

I managed to stop crying and he was quite sympathetic with me and said to take twenty minutes and then start work. I should have realised at that stage that something was not quite right with me but I didn't and just carried on as if nothing had ever happened. At the end of the week I finally got the job completed and was so glad to be out of there, as I'm sure they were to be rid of me!

I had nothing else in the pipeline work wise and when my wife rang to ask if I had any jobs to go to (we needed the money badly for the mortgage and my rent) I lied and said that I had plenty of work. My wife had always dealt with the finances and I didn't have a clue and just left it to her but now I had an ingenious plan!

Now, I'm not stupid and I know the worst thing to ever do is just rely on credit cards but something must have happened to me. All rational thoughts just went flying out the window! It was perfectly simple. I had this credit card solely in my name and it had a limit of ten thousand on it. All I had to do was draw money out each day and give the required amount to my wife to cover our debts. I kept kidding myself that work would pick up soon and I could pay back the card when it did. Needless to say, work didn't pick up and yet I kept on drawing money out and was starting not to care about how I was going to repay the debt. I would say that over the next couple of weeks, I only had about three days work. It's really surprising to think that I'd worked really hard for over twenty five years and that a strong work ethic was instilled in me but it took less than a fortnight for it to quickly ebb away.

CHAPTER 2

October 2008

No work whatsoever! I should have been earning £140 a day and working Saturdays as well, which totalled £840 for the week. I'd withdraw £300 a day, give my wife £600 a week and told her that the remaining £240 covered my rent and living expenses. In reality, I was withdrawing £1500 a week, giving my wife the £600, saving £200 towards the rent and coin operated electricity meter and keeping the remaining £700 for myself which worked out at £100 per day to do whatever I wanted with. YIPEE!!! For the next three months, my mornings consisted of going to the café immediately across the road and having scrambled eggs and smoked salmon on toast, garnished with a sprinkling of black cracked pepper (yummy!) On the extremely rare occasions that I might have a day's work, the proprietor of the above establishment would furnish me with a corned beef and pickle baguette for lunch (delish!)

If I wasn't working (which was 99% of the time) I would usually skip lunch or have something in the pub. I have a rule of not drinking in the day time so would have a coffee or coke or on the odd occasion, a pint of Guinness (hmmm, creamy!) For dinner I would have boil in the bag kippers and a slice of dry white bread to mop up the juice. The bin bag would then go immediately outside and into the wheelie bin, so it didn't stink the place out! My flat was situated between two curry houses and the one on the left had to be the finest I have ever frequented. You can only have so many boil in the bag kippers every bleedin' night and so I would treat myself to an Indian from time to time. I'd usually have just a starter and this particular dish was bloody gorgeous! King prawns (the biggest I'd ever seen) smothered in a spicy garlic sauce. The owner was a really nice bloke and he explained to me that as soon as the prawns were caught in the Indian Ocean, the fishermen would immediately put them in an ice box and the next time they were thawed out would be in his kitchen! With the dips and poppadoms you get with the meal, I found it to be more than enough. Of course, it had to be washed down with a couple of Cobras but that goes without saying! It was obviously a really good restaurant because on Friday and Saturday nights, there would be all these Bentleys and Rollers and Aston Martins, parked up outside.

When I say my place was a flat, it was actually the first in a row of five, one bedroom cottages and the landlord who owned them, lived at the end in this big house. Walking through the front door to my place, you'd be in the living room / kitchen and then there was a door which led to the downstairs toilet. That was a really good size and had plenty of cupboards, one containing the boiler, so it was nice and warm and was a good place to dry my smalls! Upstairs led directly into the bedroom, which was really big and off of that was the bathroom. The flat was less than a year old and I loved it. Because I was on the end, the wheelie bins belonging to each cottage were lined up next to where I'd park my car. I remember when my

mum came to visit, the first thing she said was, "Get the landlord to move those bins, you'll have rats!"
I never saw any, the curry house was probably using them for their dishes (ha ha)

My landlord was part of the village committee and he and all these other bigwigs would play cards down the pub each night. The first time I went in this particular pub, it reminded me of a saloon in one of those old westerns.
Around this big table, were eight men in their sixties playing cards, with my landlord at the head of the table. To me, he was the cattle baron and two of his sons were sat on stools, near the bar. As I walked in, the two sons stopped talking and stared at me and in my head, I could hear them saying, "There's a stranger in town!"
Even the music on the juke box stopped playing as I walked through the door! (Not really, I made that bit up)
That's what the village was like though. Everyone knew everyone and if someone new rode into town, the whole place would be talking. I got to know my landlord and his sons really well and they were great blokes, most of the people in the village were (after you'd been accepted that is!)
There was a Sainsbury's up the road and my first purchase was 200 fags, 24 cans of beer and a bumper pack of condoms….well, you have to think of the essentials first! Three pubs were all within easy walking (but more importantly) staggering distance from my humble abode, which was very handy. The nearest pub was right next door to the curry house and is one of the oldest drinking dens in the whole of

Essex, with some of the structure dating back 450 years! Legend has it that there's even a ghost in residence and I spoke to a couple of the regulars and they claimed to have seen it, although I doubt they could have seen much at all judging by the state they were in! I frequented this particular watering hole the first night I moved into the flat and it was a complete dump. The landlady was a right old boozer and I reckon she drank most of the profits but it did have its plus points though. To get around the smoking ban, she let the customers go upstairs to her private living space to have a cigarette and didn't mind if people stubbed their fags out on the carpet (classy lady)

I've searched on the internet and it's now a really nice restaurant / pub. I must give it a visit sometime (for research purposes you understand)

The next pub was just up the road and also had a fair bit of history behind it. The main part of the building was over 300 years old but more importantly, they had a guitarist playing live every Saturday night (right up my street!) The third pub was called The Chestnut and was the furthest away (about 3 minutes walk!) and was fairly new (only 200 years old)

It was this watering hole I chose to be my 'local'. The landlord and landlady had only recently taken over running the place and it was their first time in the pub trade. All of the locals were sceptical about whether they would last as they had 'new' ideas on how it should be run but I liked them immediately and admired the way they decided that things should be totally different. It had obviously been a very traditional English pub (in that sense I mean, no glitz or glamour) which I do like but they brought a European feel to the place. This gives you an idea of

SECTION 1: HIGH

the old time regulars: I went in on a Saturday afternoon with a book I was reading at the time and ordered a coffee and this fella at the bar complained to the landlady and said that she shouldn't serve me! I walked up to him and whispered in his ear and guess what, he never complained again....funny that?

CHAPTER 3

I got friendly with one of the old time regulars (also called John) and he lived about six paces away, so he didn't have to worry about drinking and driving (not that he could drive anyhow!) His place was so close that if he tripped out the side door of the pub (which he often did) he'd hit his head on his own front door. He was a bit of a tight git and would never offer to buy anyone a drink but he was a real old country bumkin and I loved the stories he would tell me about the village years ago. He asked me if I had been to the church down the road yet and when I told him I hadn't, he offered to show me it the next day.

"It's the oldest wooden built church in the whole bloomin' world!" he explained as I bought him a drink (again!)

John wasn't the best dressed man in the world and I think the landlady was trying to find any excuse to get him barred because he "lowered the tone" and spent an hour nursing a pint of ale while he waited for someone to buy him another.

There was a forth pub in the village but that was about ten minutes walk away and I wasn't that keen on it anyway. It was one of those pub / restaurants where couples would go to with their kids for a meal. There's nothing wrong with that but not if you're only going for a drink. All four pubs had their own darts team and the locals took it really seriously. Every Monday night, the members of each pub team would go to one of the other pubs and have a tournament. Being a new face in town, each of them asked if I would join their team but I didn't want to commit myself (someone did that for me later, ha ha)

Looking around The Chestnut of an evening, you would see all these single men with the same expression on their faces. It was something I had never noticed when I was still with my wife but now I was in the same predicament as they were. Even if they were joking and laughing, they had a pained look in their eyes as if each of them had been through a traumatic experience relationship wise. They might be laughing outside but the smile didn't seem natural somehow and I realised that I was just the same. One of these men was a tree feller (someone who cuts down trees, not a man who looks like one) and he was built like a brick shit house (or indeed………..a tree)
He had a real charisma about him, even though he kept himself mostly to himself. I've got quite a deep voice but his was so deep, it made Barry White sound like Michael Jackson. His hands were like two shovels and his shoulders, wider than the Golden Gate Bridge!
"All right John!" boomed his voice, every time he walked in. He told me that when he left his wife, he opened a small bar in Ibiza and showed me this trick he did with two wine glasses, by somehow twisting them around each other. I could never get the hang of it but was amazed how small the wine glasses looked in his gargantuan fists. Women loved him and would swoon every time he spoke but he seemed oblivious to it all, too wrapped up with his own inner demons. As I didn't have any work to go to, I was not in a rush to get home each night and so the landlord Tom and Eva

the landlady would offer me to stay behind when the pub closed and I would have a drink with them and we'd talk about ourselves and our past. Eva explained that her sister's husband had just left her and moved in with one of his secretaries. His family was in the funeral business which had been going for generations but he'd become really wealthy by having the rights to excavate entire cemeteries all over the world and relocating them if a motorway or some such thing ran through the existing land. She said that her sister would be in on the Sunday afternoon and she'd introduce me.

The next day, I picked up John in the car and we drove to the church. As we pulled up outside, I was immediately drawn under its charming spell and couldn't wait to look inside but before I did, John told me to walk round the back. We passed all these ancient grave stones and walked alongside huge oak trunks that made up the outer walls of the original part of the building. Near the end was a small inlet and when I crouched down to have a better look, I could see a small hole in the wall. Joking, I said to John, "What's this, an ancient glory hole?" (He didn't get it) "It's a leper hole," he said. "Years ago when there were lepers, they weren't allowed inside and so when it was built, they put this hole in so they could see and hear the service from outside"

I remember being blown away by that and thought to myself that it's a good job it wasn't a glory hole, otherwise my prick my fall off! We went round to the huge oak door and quietly went inside. There were jars of local handmade jam and marmalade on a small table just inside the entrance, with an honesty box next to it. If that was in London, not only would the money be gone but so would the whole fucking church and it'd end up on eBay! At the alter which was carved into the shape of an eagle, there was a very old looking bible and I asked John, "How old do you reckon that is?"

"Gawd knows!" he replied and with that, we both looked up into the rafters and burst out laughing. Walking back outside again I came upon a burial stone, under which rests a twelfth century crusader (straight up!) I mean it really was that old, not that he was buried straight up.

The main part of the church is nearly nine hundred years old and the wood is as hard as steel! My tour guide was looking decidedly parched and so we drove back into town and had a couple of drinks in The Chestnut. The weather had started to get really cold and John was nothing more than skin and bone and would shiver like mad when we where outside. I told him that I had two pairs of Long John's that I'd got from America and they even had the tailboard at the back, just like in cowboy films.

"You can have a pair if you like mate," I told him and he said that he'd love them. The next morning, I walked down to his place and hung them above the front door and then went off for some breakfast at the café. As I drove past later on, I looked over and could see these bright red pair of gandy pants, blowing in the breeze and couldn't stop laughing. I would love to have seen his face when he opened the front door to go down the pub that day.

At this stage, I was without a computer and so I joined the local library so I could use theirs. My mobile phone reception was terrible and I had to keep going outside to make or receive calls. The library was

literally next door to the pub that had the live guitarists every Saturday night and so after spending an hour on the computer each day, it seemed only natural to pop in for quick one. Lydia the lady living next door to me had split from her husband who lived about a mile down the road with their two sons who were in their late twenties. In the week, she would drink in my local and we became rather friendly (if you get my drift)
I got a phone call regarding some work and I asked her oldest son Jay if he wanted some work as a labourer and he said yes. It turned out to be another rotten job and I was getting less and less enthusiastic with my chosen profession. I liked Jay and it was awkward working with him when I was sleeping with his mum and thought it probably best not to mention it to him!

I love films and can enjoy any genre but am very particular about how well they are made. For example: "A Night to Remember" good, "Titanic" nowhere near as good. "The Treasure of the Sierra Madre" brilliant, "National Treasure" crap! Before I separated from my wife, I copied hundreds of images from my favourite films and had them printed off on an online photo company. I stuck them all up on the walls of my living room and it would make quite a talking point when anyone visited.
There was this girl who worked for the Inland Revenue (AAARRGGH!) and she was well into her films too. I brought her back one night (purely to look at my DVD collection you see) and she said, "WOW, YOU'VE GOT FREAKS! I fucking love that film!" So she couldn't have been all bad!

SECTION 1: HIGH

Laura (who owned the café I frequented every morning) was really nice and on one Sunday, I had my daughter over to visit. As I was opening the front door to my flat, Laura came over with her hands cupped together and crouched down next to my daughter. "Look what just hopped into my café," she said and when she opened her hands, a frog jumped out. We started to laugh and I told Laura that I was taking my daughter to see the old church. "Why don't you take the frog there and let him go in the field," she said. "It will be much safer there"

So that's what we did and my little girl absolutely loved the church. She bought her mum some of the homemade marmalade and was fascinated by the history of it all. She's such a clever kid and loves learning about things. Compared to her, I'm a bleedin' idiot!

On the following Saturday, I decided to pay a visit to the Tate Modern and parked my car at my brother's house and took the tube. Before I got to the Tate, I took a look around St. Pauls Cathedral (you can never get enough of a good thing) and had this feeling of being proud to be British. It's funny but since the riots of 2011, I'm now a bit ashamed to be British and wonder what the rest of the world thinks about us. All I know is this country is going steadily down the pan and something needs to be done……..fast! It wouldn't have happened in Maggie's day, I tell ya!

I'd never been to an art gallery before in my life which is crazy because I love art. I'd spent most of my adult life working six or seven days a week and so didn't have the time or I couldn't afford it. People would say to me that it was free to go to certain museums or galleries but I literally didn't have enough for the train fare. All of my salary would go on bills in one form or another and there just wasn't anything left over for leisure activities. I was absolutely blown away by the Tate Modern (you were right bruv) and spent about four hours of bliss looking at all the works of art. Something weird happened to me while I was there and I'm not sure why. As I'm absorbing all of these paintings and sculptures, I realised that I was starting to get an erection and I had to stand up close to the paintings on the wall so no one would notice. It sounds funny now but at the time I was quite worried and didn't understand what was going on. It's not as if I was looking at erotic images or anything like that and I felt that I'd better leave (once me cock had shrunk down again that is!)

On reflection, I think that because it was my first visit to an art gallery and I was on my own and therefore could take my time and look at what I wanted and for how long I wanted, my brain had some kind of overload or something. I still don't really know why it happened because I definitely wasn't feeling horny? On the way out, I went into the gift shop and bought myself one of those wooden hands that can be manipulated into different positions: artists use them to sketch with. Before getting on the tube, I popped into a pub for a Guinness and joked around with these three Polish girls working behind the bar by putting the wooden hand in all different types of rude positions.

CHAPTER 4

My nephew Steve came up from Hampshire to visit one Saturday and we planned to go for a curry and then a drink. I had to pick him up from Epping station and as I turned the corner and drove down the hill to the entrance, he jumped out in the road and started pulling a stupid face. At that moment, I noticed two really fit looking girls out of the corner of my eye, walking up the hill. I was so busy staring at them that I didn't realise Steve hadn't gotten out of the way and so consequently, I run him over.

He bounced off the bonnet of the car and landed on his back, in the middle of the road. My first concern of course, was to see if the two girls had noticed (I thought that if they'd seen me run someone over, it might cramp my style!) Looking around, I could see they were giggling and when I turned back I saw Steve standing up again, laughing his head off.

He opened the passenger door and said, "Let's get the fuck out of here!"

There was this big group of people waiting to be picked up, looking on with a mixture of horror and bewilderment.

"Did you see those two birds?" I asked him.

"You nearly fucking killed me!"

"Yeh but, you should have seen 'em!"

"What about me? I could be dead!"

"Look, look, there they are!" I yelled and pointed to the couple of beauties as they were just about to turn the corner.

"Fuck me! Yeh, they are fit, aren't they!" he replied.

He then opened his window, stuck the top part of his body out and yelled, "Oi! All right, you old slags!"

It took about twenty minutes to drive back to my place and I nearly crashed the car about ten times because we were laughing so much. I can't remember what we were talking about but it must have been good. As soon as we walked through the door, Steve opened the fridge and started laughing. All that was in there were forty eight cans of beer and a packet of kippers. He threw me a can, had one for himself and I put some music on nice and loud. We began dancing around the living room and then started to hear this banging on the wall, coming from next door and Steve looked over at me.

"She likes it really," I said, "she's probably got a hang over"

A short while later I gave Steve a mini tour of the village and he really liked it. I was going to show him the church but when I suggested it, he said, "Fuck that! Let's go back and have a drink!"

So after several more cans, we decided to get ready and headed off into the night.

We started off in The Chestnut for a couple or four, where I introduced him to Tom and Eva and we both agreed that we'd have a curry when we'd finished our beverages. On our way to the restaurant, I suggested that we have a quick drink in the really old pub but ended up staying for about five beers. Some people I'd gotten to know said that they were going to a pub about three miles away and did we want to share a cab. Steve looked at me and we decided that we'd have our meal later on. After about four more beers at this new pub, we thought that we'd better have

something to eat and so ordered a packet of crisps. We ate about half the pack between us and feeling rather bloated, discarded them and carried on drinking. We eventually ended up back at the old pub next to where I lived, for some afterhours liquid refreshment and carried on with our drinkfest. At about 3am, Steve said that he was knackered and so I gave him my key and told him to leave it under the bin outside my front door, so I could get in myself and then carried on drinking to about six before finally retiring for the evening. I got home and the sofa bed was half constructed with bits of it strewn all over the place and when I went upstairs, the big oaf was sprawled across my bed snoring his head off.
"Marvellous!"
I managed to budge the brute over slightly and crashed out next to him with my clothes still on.

Steve woke me up at 10am and said that he had to catch the eleven o'clock train, so I had a quick cuppa, brushed my teeth and drove him to the station which was about five miles away. We said our goodbyes and I drove back home, feeling wide awake and ready for another session. Going indoors briefly, I made my bed, reconstructed the sofa bed and then tidied up a bit before heading back to my local booze emporium. Although it was October, the weather was glorious and there was not a cloud in the sky. I was still wearing the same clothes I had on the night before and as I arrived outside the pub, there were loads of people sitting outside in the sun. All of these classic cars kept driving past, bibbing their hooters and it felt like the middle of summer. There was this biker with a Harley parked up outside and it was a work of art, smothered in chrome gothic characters and skeletons! He'd replaced the headlamp with a full-size skull made from chrome and the two lights shined out of the empty eye sockets. I could have spent hours looking at it; there wasn't one inch of the bike that didn't have something cool to look at. Even the footrest was in the shape of a clawed hand. I spent about twenty minutes talking to him and about another five, trying to get into the pub because it was so busy outside with people blocking the entrance. When I walked inside it was packed to the rafters, probably to do with the olive and carrot dips at the bar. Mr. "Don't serve the coffee drinker" didn't look happy because the place was full of all these well to do people and I was immediately uplifted by his misery! I forced my way through the throng of people and up to the bar, where eventually Eva served me. She introduced me to her sister Eleanor who was perched on a stool by the bar and half way towards getting pissed. John was ingratiating himself with her and her family, so he could get loads of drinks for nothing and I had a go at playing darts with Eleanor's daughter. She was really attractive and all of the single men with the melancholy faces were drooling at the mouth (me included!)

So I'd been out since seven the previous night, had four hours uncomfortable sleep, shared half a packet of crisps and was back on it boozing. By now I was getting on really well with the landlady's family (all doctors and lawyers and stuff) but then I needed a piss. As I walked away, I squeezed Eleanor's arm in a friendly/flirting manner and left her trying to understand John's country accent while he impressed her family with tales of derring-do. They were all

SECTION 1: HIGH

wearing what you could tell were very expensive clothes and John had on this old green cardigan, covered in moth holes. When I got back, there was another beer waiting for me and I sank it in no time at all. I don't know what was up with me that day but I was able to keep on drinking. By about 7pm, I'd completely lost track of what day it was, let alone the time. Eleanor and her family had left a couple of hours earlier and now, the usual evening drinkers starting coming in. Eva made me eat some food and kept telling me to get some sleep but I wouldn't listen and didn't leave for home until closing time at eleven that night.

I think I must have slept through the whole of Monday and was ready for more liquor on the Tuesday. Back down to the local that night and Eleanor was there again, on her own this time. She'd obviously been going through a difficult time with her husband leaving and was getting slowly drunk. Tom and Eva were talking to us in between serving customers and John was in his usual corner, drinking his beer as slowly as possible in the hope that someone would buy him another. I excused myself and went to the toilet and was minding my own business (and holding it too!) when Eleanor walked in. I was washing my hands and she grabbed hold of me and started groping and kissing me all over. I returned the compliment and then she said, "I must get back to the bar before she gets suspicious," and handed me her mobile number. Surprised but pleasantly so, I went out into the back courtyard and had a cigarette and stored her number into my phone. When I returned to the bar, she was in conversation with her brother-in-law Tom and so to

BIPOLAR…..ME?

play it cool I had a game of darts with John, saying to him, "Loser buys the next round"
"What? What? How'd ya mean?" he panicked.
"Only joking John….you can get the next two in"
"Eh?"
Out of the corner of my eye, I saw Eleanor get up and say that she had to go. When she walked by, heading for the front door, she whispered to me, "Call me"
I finished the game of darts as quickly as possible, not caring if John beat me (I bought his next pint anyway) and then said that I had to be going home. Walking back to my flat, I rang Eleanor and she gave me the directions to her house. Grabbing a few beers and a bottle of wine I had in the fridge, I got in the car and headed to Eleanor's place. It was in the middle of nowhere and I had to give her another call as I was driving down this narrow country lane but eventually I found it. We forgot all about the wine and beer and just got down to business and the next morning, I took a shower in this massive wet room. The house was on acres and acres of land and had its own stables for the horses that pull the funeral carriages along. Eleanor said that she had to get to work but would see me down the pub in a couple of days' time. When I got home, there was a load of mail waiting for me. One of the letters was from the credit card company demanding payment (I threw that in the bin) and another was from a different credit card company, asking if I wanted to apply for a new one. There was also a note from my neighbour which simply read: I missed you last night John boy x
(It actually said big boy but I felt silly saying it. Her glasses were obviously way too strong for her….not that she wore any)

SECTION 1: HIGH

I put the note on the shelf next to the artist's wooden hand, which today was making a peace sign. I'd maxed out on my existing card and decided to apply for the new one. They agreed and in a matter of days, I had £10,000 again (it was a miracle!)
Later that day, my mobile rang and it was my mum asking if her and dad could come and visit.
"Of course you can," I replied. "it will be great to see you," and then we arranged for them to stay on the following Saturday evening. I'm naturally a tidy person anyway but made a mental note to give the flat an extra special clean before they arrived. The phone rang again and it was a guy I'd done work for on properties he had on his books as a letting agent. He asked me if I could do some tiling in his own bathroom and I told him that I'd come round and have a look tomorrow. I had initially gotten to know him by laying some decking at his own house, where my two sons helped me and they were really useful. I only had to tell them something once and they picked it up straight away. I remember on that particular job, I was firing four inch nails into the four by two joists with a nail gun, when one of the nails must of hit a knot in the wood and caused it to bend back round and go through my finger and out of my nail. Luckily, the force of it pushed my hand away and so it wasn't left stuck in my finger. I really wanted to get to a particular stage on the job for that day and so I got some kitchen towel and wrapped it round my finger and held it in place with some electrical tape and then carried on, occasionally spilling drops of blood on the plush new decking.
That night in the pub and after everyone else had left; I was having a quiet drink with Tom and Eva and

telling them about all the decking jobs I'd done. Tom explained to me about Eleanor's house and how she had this vast amount of decking out the back. I was thinking to myself, "I know, I was drinking a cup of coffee on it this morning!"

The next day and I went to see the property letting guy. He was a really nice bloke and so easy to get along with. He showed me what needed doing in the bathroom and said that he'd get all the materials for the following Monday. On the way home, I decided to try a different pub that evening and opted for the one with the live music on a Saturday night.

CHAPTER 5

The barman on that particular night was a guy called Josh, who was in his early twenties. We got on really well and he said that when the pub shut that evening, he and some mates were going to a nightclub and would I like to go along? I said that I'd love to and so when Josh finished his shift, we got in his car and he floored it all down these country lanes to the next big town where the club was. It's quite a well known nightclub and features a lot in one of those crap reality T.V shows. I couldn't believe how packed it was for a week day and loved the way it was set out. It reminded me of a labyrinth with all of these corridors going off in different directions and had fish tanks built into the walls. Each corridor had its own bar and seating space in the middle and they all led to the main area in the centre of the building which housed the dance floor.
Outside there was a central courtyard and the downstairs bar had its own D.J with an intimate room containing these giant sofas running around the walls. While I was having a cigarette outside, Josh pointed to this girl and asked if I recognised her. It was one of those C list celebrities and she clearly loved herself and the attention she was getting. Behind where she stood, there was this really cool looking statue of a Buddha and so I went up closer to her and loud enough so she could hear me I said, "Wow Josh, look!"
She gazed in my direction with an arrogant smirk on her face and saw me pointing in her direction as I

walked right up to her and called out to Josh, "Man, I love that statue!"

You could tell she was fuming and so I turned to her and said, "It's you! I'm star struck!"

She started to giggle and said, "No you're not"

I smiled at her and replied, "You're right, I'm not" and walked away.

I've since found out that she has had some mental health issues in her own life and is as screwed up as I am and feel a bit bad about it now.

Upstairs by the main dance floor and opposite the D.J, was a guy playing the bongos in time with the beat of the tune that was playing. He had a microphone rigged up next to the drums, so the sound was coming out of the speakers. I really appreciate anyone who can play a musical instrument well and he was bloody brilliant!

While Josh and his mates got up on the podium to dance, I went for a drink and was talking to the girl behind the bar. This black bloke was standing next to me and so I got talking to him too. He explained that he was a medical student from Africa and was over here doing his studies. I found it difficult understanding what he was saying, what with his strong accent and the loud music and so I told him I was going outside to the courtyard for a cigarette. He followed me and when we were in the open air, I immediately realised that he was gay by the way he was dressed (a bright purple shirt with silver buttons) and his mannerisms. While we were talking, he kept touching my arm and so I told him to stop and explained that I wasn't that way inclined. He kept on doing it and so I walked away and went upstairs again but he started following me. As I was about to walk into the main dance floor area, these two bouncers were dragging this bloke out and he was covered in blood. There was a big struggle and so I pushed the black guy out the way, so he didn't get hurt. I remember thinking back to that incident and laughing to myself that I'd protected him as if he were my girlfriend. Making my way to the bar with him still in tow, I bought myself another beer and had to tell him to leave me alone. He went off to the toilet and I made my escape and pushed myself through the packed dance floor and up to the podium. Seeing as I'm getting on a bit, Josh had to pull me up onto the bloody thing and we all carried on dancing. After the club shut, we went to the car park and Josh's friends got in their cars and I climbed into Josh's car. Being kids, they drove like maniacs down these country roads and I felt nervous because you could tell they didn't have much experience but luckily I made it home in one piece!

Friday morning and I went to Sainsbury's to stock up on supplies for my mum and dad's visit on the Saturday. I remember walking around the store at 100mph, like a man on a mission and my mind was racing all over the place. I'd bought a notepad and started to write myself memos about the most insignificant things, such as: "Flush the toilet" or "Eat something" or "Have one hour's sleep"
I then went to the library and wrote a couple of emails to family members. I'm not sure what they were about but they were sure to be the ravings of a lunatic and only fuelled my family's concern for me. Heading back to the flat, I was full of energy so I did fifty push ups and fifty sit ups. I still had loads of energy and stuck some music on and danced around the place

while doing the housework. Lunchtime and I popped over to Josh's pub and had a Guinness, then went out the back for a cigarette and there was this guy dealing coke to some fella I didn't recognise. They'd never seen me before and tried to hide what they were doing and I pretended not to notice but every now and then, I couldn't help but give the dealer dirty looks. I don't have a problem with people taking drugs, as long as they are old enough, it's their choice. It's some of the dealers I can't stand. Back inside the pub and I started talking to Wendy the landlady who claimed to be a white witch! I decided not to tell her about the goings on out the back and asked who was on tomorrow night for the guitar evening.

"Steve Forward" she replied.

"Shit, I'm gonna miss him because I've got my mum and dad staying!"

"Why don't you bring them along?"

"They don't like loud music and wouldn't appreciate it"

The tree feller from The Chestnut walked in and ordered a pint.

"All right mate!" I called out to him, "what you doing here? Did they run out of beer at The Chestnut?"

He strolled over to me, not looking too happy.

"I've been barred," he said.

"What for?"

"I just snapped and started throwing chairs around the place"

"Why? What's the matter?"

"My fucking wife man! She won't let me see the kids"

For someone so big and strong, I looked at his face and saw the expression of a really vulnerable human being. I felt so sorry for him.

SECTION 1: HIGH

We had a few beers together (so much for not drinking in the day) and I tried lifting his spirits and when we finally left, he seemed a bit more cheerful.

Back at the flat at about 2pm and I set my alarm to go off at 5pm and then went to sleep. A load of weird dreams flooded my mind and I woke up in a cold sweat with the alarm bleeping in my ears. I'd completely lost my bearings and because it was dark outside, I thought it was the following morning. Turning to look at the clock, I was relieved to see that it was still Friday (I really fancied going back to the white witch's pub that night as it was Karaoke evening and was sure to be busy) Getting dressed and leaving the flat, I went back to Sainsbury's and bought my kippers and some thick chocolate milkshake as a guy had told me it helped prevent a hangover because it lined the stomach. I then went to the cash point and drew out £300. Back at the flat and I stuck some music on nice and loud and could just about hear Lydia next door, clapping her hands in time with the tune. I would play C.D's on my DVD player and through the home cinema system and in the four months I lived in the flat, I never watched T.V once. About a week after moving in, I got a letter from the T.V licensing people, asking me to pay my bill and so I wrote to them and explained that I didn't watch television and only watched DVD's and therefore should be exempt from paying. Everyone I told said that I would have to pay but I got a letter back saying I didn't and so I got it framed and hung it above the T.V. It wasn't about the money; it was about having to pay to watch all of that reality T.V crap that had taken over the airwaves! After I'd eaten my beloved kippers and washed up, I went upstairs for a full head shave and a shower and

then got dressed up in some fancy duds. The pub was packed and Laura (the café owner) was singing "Back to Black" by Amy Winehouse. She had a great voice and I was well impressed! The white witch's daughter Zoe and her boyfriend, with whom I became mates with, were singing next and everyone joined in and it was a great atmosphere. A short while later, I went out the back for a smoke and the drug dealer recognised me from earlier on.
"Alright baldy" he said in a joking manner.
I forced a smile, nodded and then got as far away from him as possible for the rest of the night.

CHAPTER 6

Saturday morning and another gloriously sunny day. It was the end of October and really warm. My mum and dad were due to arrive in two hours, that gave me enough time to change the sheets and put a wash on in the communal laundry room at the end of the row of flats. These were coin operated also and the unspoken rule was to always have a pound credit in the washer and dryer as an emergency back up and I had just enough time to run the vacuum cleaner round before they knocked on the front door. It was great to see them both as it had been about four months since I'd seen them last and they really liked the flat. After a cup of tea and a chat, I offered to show them around the village and couldn't resist starting off by taking them to the old church. Like me, they loved it and my dad couldn't get his head round how old it was. I then took them to another church just off the main road and two minutes walk from my flat. Inside, there was a plaque on the wall that described the Father of the church in 1912. He had been invited over to New York to assist in his brother's marriage and booked a passage on the Titanic. Witnesses claimed that he helped women and children onto life boats and refused many attempts by crew members, to save himself. Needless to say, the poor sod went down with the tub! When we got back to the flat, my mum discovered that I hardly had any pots and pans (or food) and so treated me to some.

That evening we went down to The Chestnut for a drink and Eleanor was in there with her daughter and her boyfriend. We had a really good night and I obviously kept it quiet about me and Eleanor's adventures! My dad got drunk but was in really good spirits (and some really good spirits were in him!)
Not feeling the least bit tired, when we got back to the flat, my mum and dad went upstairs to bed and I went to the witch's pub for a few more drinks.
The next morning and my dad was suffering a bit but said what a good night he'd had. Mum made us a full English and copious cups of tea and that seemed to put him on the right track again. We said our goodbyes and I promised I would visit them in Hampshire soon.

After they had left, I decided to give The Chestnut another visit and it was absolutely packed! Eleanor was there with her family again and she asked if I would like to go back with them for Sunday lunch.
"Yeah, I'd love to"
It seemed a bit weird sitting round the dining table with this woman about fifteen years older than me and her daughter and boyfriend but they didn't seem fussed and it wasn't as weird as the fact there was a human leg bone propped up against the wall next to us! Eleanor explained that the warehouse where they usually stored all of the remains of an excavated cemetery had problems with its lease and so as a temporary measure, they'd had to bring all of the earth and remains back to her house.
"There's a huge pile of earth and bones in the back garden" she explained, "We can go and have a rummage around after lunch if you like?"

SECTION 1: HIGH

"Yeh, why not?"
After we had eaten (not spare ribs I'm pleased to say) the daughter and the boyfriend said they had to go off to some polo match or something and so me and Eleanor went into the back garden and climbed this mountain of earth. She had about nine acres of land, so it was stuck in the middle of the lawn. Every now and then, she would find a bone and tell me from which part of the corpse it came from. She sure knew her way around a body (dead or alive!)

Monday night down the witch's pub and Josh was on bar duty. It was pretty quiet in there and me and Josh were talking about comics and what were our favourites. I told him that I'd once made a comic twenty years earlier and he said that he'd love to see it and so I finished my drink and said to him I'll be back in a minute before returning to my flat to get it. It was made in 1990 and is full of references to all my favourite films. The drawings are crude but I wanted to get it finished as soon as possible and even then, it took just over a year to complete. Back at the pub and I showed Josh my "masterpiece" and he absolutely loved it!
"Did you really do this?" he asked. "I love the fact that it's all done by hand!"
"Well I didn't do it with me bleedin' feet, did I boy!"
Times sure had changed since I was his age; everything was done on computers nowadays. He lifted up the bar hatch and went round to the other customers with the comic in his hand saying, "He did this, he did this. It's bloody brilliant!"
I was still unaware that I was suffering from bipolar and hearing his complimentary words got me thinking

it really was as good as he thought. I was starting to get thirsty and asked Josh to get back behind the ramp and serve me and as he closed the hatch behind him he said, "Oi mate, you've got to get this published!"

I explained that I'd thought about it years ago but it would have cost too much money to get it printed up en masse. He asked me if he could borrow it and I agreed but told him to look after it. To me, it wasn't a comic but the film I had always wanted to direct. It's funny how you change as you get older. When I made it all those years ago, it was all about violence and action but now I'd love to make a movie that didn't have either but could still be really enthralling. Some of the customers were starting to get a bit annoyed with Josh because instead of serving them, he had his head stuck in the comic and it was at that precise moment I had my "Eureka" moment! Maybe I <u>could</u> get it published but not in printed form. I asked Josh if he knew anyone who designed websites and he said that one of his best mates ran his own business from his bedroom at his mum's house.

My idea was to set up a website where people could subscribe in instalments to read the comic and I could edit it in such a way that when they reached the end of each instalment, I'd leave it on a cliff hanger so they'd come back for more. That was the easy part. The tricky part was going to be able to raise the funds to get it copyrighted for the entire planet!

(Since having this book published, I realise it is much easier to do now than it was back then and doesn't cost much at all)

I told Josh to arrange a meeting with his website designer mate Alex for the following day and then said that I wanted to go back to that nightclub again. I was full of energy and had to get rid of it somehow.

"It's shut tonight mate" he told me, "but there's another one that's almost as good!"

"Are you up for it?" I asked him

"I can't tonight; I promised I'd see my girlfriend after work"

"Shit! Would you drop me off there and I'll make my own way back?"

"I would do mate but she'll moan if I'm late"

"I'll cut you in on the comic if I make it rich!" I explained

"It's a deal!"

Josh dropped me off out the front and I went inside. It was a Monday night and absolutely rammed! I walked up to the nearest bar and got myself a drink, with my head swimming with ideas on how to get some more money for my brilliant idea! After another beer I went to the toilet and saw a bloke dealing dope (what was it with that area? It was like the fucking Bronx!)

Back at the bar and the girl serving asked why I was shaking my head. I said something like, "It's terrible nowadays, you can't go anywhere without people taking drugs" (I sound like my dad) and she asked me what I meant.

"There's a bloke dealing dope in the toilets" I said and walked off, thinking no more about it. About ten minutes later, these three bouncers walked up to me and asked me to go with them to this room out the back. I didn't have a fucking clue what was going on.

"Can you show us which one is the drug dealer?" one of them asked.

"No way!" I replied, realising the bar girl must have told them what I'd said. Even though I'm no fan of

drug dealers, I wasn't about to grass the bloke up. It's different if he was selling it to school kids or something but this was in a nightclub where you might expect to see something like that. The biggest bouncer put his hand on my shoulder and said, "We have a very strict drugs policy here and anyone found using them on the premises is automatically barred for life"
"Sorry mate, I still can't help you out" I replied.
"If you don't tell us then you'll be banned too!"
There was no way I was going to get slung out for something I didn't do and so reasoned with him.
"I'll point him out but don't want you going up to him with me stood next to you!"
"Okay, now show us where he is"
"I don't want you near me, keep your distance and I'll nod to you when I see him"
So I went off in search of this bloke and could see the bouncers following me from afar. I finally spotted the bloke upstairs, sitting round a table with a load of mates and I walked up to him and said, "Alright mate?"
He looked at me a bit suspicious and said, "Who wants to fucking know?"
"Such awful manners!" I thought to myself, "This prick deserves everything he gets!"
"You might wanna get up and follow me, you won't want your mates seeing," I told him.
"What the fuck are you talking about, you cunt?" he so eloquently replied. With that, I walked round the corner and pointed him out to the three bouncers. I decided it best if I left myself as I didn't want to run into any of his mates and made a mental note, not to go there again! Part of me hated doing what I did but he was a total wanker, so who gives a fuck!

CHAPTER 7

The next morning and I realised I was going to have to get a computer if I wanted to be serious about my comic idea. It just wouldn't be practical going to the library every day and in any case, they only let you use it for an hour a time. I rang my eldest son and asked him what was the best laptop I could get for about £500 and he gave me the info I needed. I drew some more money out, bought the laptop and went to another store and purchased a scanner and some speakers (I might as well listen to something while I'm working!)

I then rushed back to the flat, set the laptop and scanner up and made myself a cup of coffee (extra strong, I needed to stay awake!)

I'd just started taking a sip of the coffee when my phone rang. It made me jump and I spilled the whole cup all over the keyboard.

"FUCK IT!"

I answered the phone, "HELLO!"

"Hi John, its Josh. You okay?"

"I've just bought the most expensive laptop I can afford and I've spilled coffee all over the fucker!"

"Oh, is it gonna be all right?" he asked.

"Well it's still going but the keys are a bit sticky" I replied.

Josh told me that he'd arranged a meeting with Alex (the website guy) for 4pm. I told him to come round to mine and we'd go there together and spent the next hour cleaning up the laptop and table and the

instruction book (which I had to put on the radiator to dry out).
It was a brand new book but now looked like a piece of ancient parchment. The weather was really warm outside and I was sweating like a pig with the heating on and so changed into a pair of shorts.
Once I'd got the computer looking half decent, I started looking up companies that dealt with copyright issues and found one in London that specialised in the subject. I called the number on the website and was put through to this guy who started giving me the basic information I needed to know money wise. The problem of putting the comic online was that if it hasn't got a copyright, then anyone can copy it themselves and then share it with other people or even claim it to be their own work. This guy told me that I could have it copyrighted in the U.K for free but the problem is that anyone in the world would be able to see it on the website and then they could have it for themselves. To cover the entire planet, including North and South America and Australasia, it would come to about £20,000. I remember not being fazed by this one bit and was immediately thinking that I would have to apply for more credit cards! I arranged to have a meeting with this guy and some of his colleagues, the next day (Little did I know that a few years later, all of this could be achieved online for a fraction of the cost, forty quid to be precise)
4pm
Josh arrived and looked at me a bit strange because I was wearing just a pair of shorts, so I turned off the heating, got changed and we went to see Alex. I was expecting someone in a suit to answer the door but

instead, this middle aged woman opened the door, smiled and then shouted upstairs, "Alex, it's for you!"
"Alright mum!" came the reply.
Alex came down the stairs in his pyjamas and some big furry slippers that looked like a pair of monster's hairy feet and I looked at Josh who gave me a reassuring nod. We all sat down in the living room and Alex's mum came in with the tea and biscuits. Since speaking to the copyright guy, I'd fine tuned my idea and explained it to Alex and Josh. Not only could people subscribe to read my comic, they could also have their own comics placed on the website and 'our team of highly trained professionals' could polish it up for them by changing the text or adding colours etc. We could even add voices to the images and really bring their creations to life! Alex said it would be much cheaper if I scanned the pages of my comic, rather than pay for him to do it.
I said I was already on the case! Most of the pages were made up of six boxes of drawings and there were one hundred and twenty pages in total. Some of the text had mistakes crossed out and Alex suggested that they could be erased but Josh disagreed and said, "That's what makes it so good, the fact that it's not perfect!"
I could see his reasoning and agreed with him to keep the mistakes and then thought my comic could be used as an example to people wanting their own comics displayed on the website. They could see a before and after on mine, with all of the mistakes corrected and the dialogue written in typed font. The idea was to split each instalment up into ten pages. When the subscriber viewed each page, they could click on each box and it would expand to fill the whole screen. With

six boxes per page, that meant each instalment would consist of sixty boxes. We thought for a while on how much should be charged for each instalment and settled on twenty five pence. Alex thought it should be one pound but I was determined it should be as cheap as possible. I told him that the subscriber shouldn't be able to copy the pages and forward them to someone else and he said he could do that.

Just say ten thousand people subscribed and they read the whole thing, at twenty five pence per instalment of ten pages, multiplied by twelve to total one hundred and twenty pages. That worked out to thirty thousand pounds. Type the word "comic" into Google and you'll get over four hundred million results. Alex was pretty confident he could get me on page one with the word "comic", so it was looking more than likely that over ten thousand people would show an interest. There was one big problem though that had to be sorted before I could put my comic out there on the internet. Back in the seventies, there was a British comic called "Bullet" whose main character was called just "Fireball". He was raised by his uncle, Lord Peter Flint aka Warlord, after his parents, who worked for British Intelligence, were killed in a mysterious car crash.
Warlord was a comic in its own right and Bullet ran from 1976-79 then was merged with Warlord. As a kid, I loved the Fireball character and started to make my own small comics with him as the hero. I gave him a first name and forgot all about the Warlord connection and more importantly, cranked up the violence! These mini-comics I made were only about three or four pages long and my sister Jane kept saying

SECTION 1: HIGH

to me that I should make a longer one and so I finally decided to do just that, to get it out of my system. The problem I faced now was the name Fireball, it was all over my comic and I had to change it so I didn't get done for breach of copyright.

In the village where I lived, there was this window cleaner guy called Darren Allen who was I'm guessing in his early thirties, with learning difficulties and had the mental capacity of a ten year old. Whenever you'd drive through the village, Darren would always be there, either cleaning windows or sitting on a bench by himself. I asked people about him and they said his parents would make him leave the house early in the morning and tell him not to come home until the evening. Everyone said he was a great guy but sometimes I would hear people taking the piss out of him when they were drunk. Josh told me that Darren was in the pub over the road one night and he accidently spilt this bloke's beer. He was very apologetic but the guy hit him so hard, he broke his jaw and then him and his mates just stood there laughing as he lay on the floor. I became friends with Darren and thought it would be a good idea if I changed Fireball's name to his but that would take a lot of work as the word Fireball was everywhere in my comic!

"Wouldn't it be great," I thought to myself, "If the name Darren Allen became known all over the world. That would make his day!"

Although Fireball's name was going to be changed to Darren's, the two couldn't have been more different. Fireball (my Fireball, not the original 70's Fireball) was 5, 10" with a slim muscular physique, a lovely mop of thick black hair and a moustache, whereas

Darren was about 6, 2", seventeen stone and had long scraggly, ginger brown hair, tied in a pony tail. Fireball would always wear an Armani jacket; Darren would always wear a donkey jacket. Fireball, the finest Italian leather boots; Darren, a pair of steel toe caps. The only thing they had in common was the fact they both sported a rather dandy moustache but Darren's was all shredded wheat looking as opposed to Fireball's illustrious thick, dark tash. In Josh's pub, the chef who made the lunches was pretty handy with a computer (his pies weren't bad either) and so I decided to approach him regarding the change of name required to get my comic rolling. So now I had the website being constructed, a meeting arranged with the copyright guy and a new name for my main character. I was feeling good and suggested to Josh that we hit a nightclub after he finished work that evening. When I got back to the flat at about 6pm, I changed the wooden hand from a peace sign to a "Thumbs Up"

I realised that I didn't have much money for the night as I'd used it all up on the laptop and scanner and so I rang Eleanor to see if she could lend me some until the following day (when I could draw out some more!)

She said that she would meet me in The Chestnut at 8pm and that left me a couple of hours to start scanning the comic.

CHAPTER 8

7:30pm
"Shit, I need to get ready!"
I'd only scanned about twenty pages, it was taking ages but I had to stop and have a shave and shower. I put some smart clothes on and walked down to the pub to meet Eleanor. Before I went in, I saw John out the front smoking a roll-up and we had a talk for a couple of minutes. Eleanor's brother-in-law Tom must have seen me through the window and came outside.
"John, can I have a word with you in private?" he said. He had a serious expression on his face and I was confused! We walked round the side and he said, "Eleanor rang me about an hour ago and asked to borrow some money"
"Shit!" I thought, "I know where this is going!"
"I asked her what it was for," he continued, "and she said she needed it to lend to you. I don't appreciate you sleeping with my sister-in-law and then trying to get money out of her"
"It's not like that," I replied but he cut me short.
"I think it's best if you don't drink here for a while" he said.
"But Tom"
"You heard what I said"
"Am I barred?" I asked.
"No, you're not barred, I just think it's best you don't come in here for the time being"
"I'm sorry Tom," I replied and walked away with my tail between my legs and felt terrible because I really

liked Tom and Eva and the last thing I wanted to do was upset them.

I needed cheering up but only had twenty quid on me and so walked over to the witch's pub and ordered a beer off Josh. He could tell something was wrong but I didn't go into the details of what had just happened, I just said that I had a headache and was going home. Back at the flat and the wooden hand made the "Thumbs Down" position. It was only 9 o'clock and I couldn't draw any more money out until midnight. I decided to carry on with the scanning in the meantime and managed to get the whole lot finished by eleven thirty. This cheered me up and I changed the hand to the O.K gesture. I was starting to get the urge for some female company and so got a cab to the nearest nightclub, which I reached at 12:05am and walked over the road to the cash point and drew out £300. It was a pretty uneventful evening and I still had the urge for, "you know what!"

A taxi took me back home at 2am and I was desperate for a shag! I'd never been with a hooker before but thought the time was right and decided to call another cab to take me into London. When the cabbie picked me up at 3am, he looked surprised that I wanted to be taken to Leicester Square. My plan was to go to Stringfellows and ask around if anyone knew a decent knocking shop and I shared all of this information with the driver! We pulled up at the taxi rank outside Stringfellows at 3:45am and it was closing up but there was still a bouncer on the door. I told the cabbie to wait for me and walked up to the bouncer, who was looking at me all suspicious like.

"Do you know where I can get a decent brass?" I asked him.

This huge black man didn't even look at me and didn't say anything either. All of a sudden, this drunk staggered up to us and started mouthing off to the bouncer. I looked at him with my hardest stare (I learnt that from Paddington Bear) and told him to, "Fuck off!"

It's more likely that he did fuck off due to the presence of the bouncer but I didn't really care, at least he was gone. The cab driver was looking at me from his car with a worried expression on his face and I gave him a reassuring nod. A funny thing happened then. The bouncer turned to me and told me to hang on while he made a phone call. I can only assume that he was willing to help me now because I'd told the drunk to fuck off.

He got out his mobile phone and made a call to someone and when he hung up, told me to wait ten minutes. I then walked back over to my mini cab driver and told him to keep waiting (I wasn't letting him go anywhere until I felt that everything was okay) and about five minutes later this other mini cab pulled up behind my one. The driver got out and walked over to the bouncer, who whispered something in his ear. This cab driver then told me to get in his car and I weighed him up and immediately felt safe with him (I can't explain why)

I finally told the other cab driver that he could go and as I was paying him, he said, "Be careful John"

For his trouble, I gave the bouncer a score and got in the other cab and asked where we were going.

"Paddington," (no, not that one) he replied in a thick African accent.

We got chatting on the way and he told me that he used to be a bouncer too but what with the recession, work had become really scarce and so he took up mini cab driving to make ends meet. He lived with his wife and two kids who went to college over here and sent money home to his parents when he could. I asked him if he'd tried any doormen work in the Essex area and he explained that he'd made a few calls but to no avail so I said that if I ever went to any nightclubs near me, I'd ask them if they were looking for registered doormen.

We eventually arrived at our destination and pulled into a cobbled mews where he parked up and we walked up to the side door of this Victorian townhouse. Inside and we climbed a steep flight of stairs to the first floor and walked into a kitchen come dining room where there were two young men and two girls, all working on their laptops. My driver said hello and then went and made himself a cup of coffee and told me that I had to choose one of the girls. Bearing in mind I had never done this sort of thing before, I felt a little bit embarrassed but decided to go with this girl with blonde hair, although both of them were stunning. The cab driver said, "I will wait here for you John and drop you to the station afterwards"

The girl got up from the table and took me by the hand up a second flight of stairs to the next floor where there was this older woman sitting on a sofa on the landing, reading a book. She told me that I had one hour and then she would knock on the bedroom door. It turned out that they were all students from Poland and the girls did this for some extra cash. When we got in the bedroom, I was feeling ultra paranoid about being ripped off and told her that I needed to use the bathroom but in reality; I wanted to stick the money I

SECTION 1: HIGH

had in my sock and then stuff the sock in one of my shoes. It turned out that I needn't have worried and they were all good people and the girl in question was really good! The cabbie did wait for me like he'd said and as I was being driven to the station; he told me that he used their services now and again and I promised to ring him if I found anything out workwise before saying goodbye. On the train home and all of the commuters must have thought I was mad because I was sitting there daydreaming, with a big smile on my face! I eventually got home at about 8am and went to Laura's café for some breakfast before crashing out in my bed for about four hours. At least I'd found a way to use up some of that energy!

CHAPTER 9

My alarm went off at 1pm and I got up and had a shower before ringing a cab to take me to the meeting with the copyright guy in London. When the cab arrived, I jumped in the front, clutching onto my comic and explained to the driver that it could make me a millionaire! I'd clearly lost the plot by this stage and really did think my website idea was going to make me rich and even looked into getting a safe deposit box because I thought the comic would be so valuable! It would have cost me £200 a month.

"No problem!" I thought and must have sounded convincing telling the driver my ingenious plan because he bought right into it, saying the website was a brilliant idea and when he dropped me off, he wished me the best of luck. (I'm not sure he would have been so enthusiastic if I'd actually shown him the comic!)

I walked inside this building and the receptionist told me to take a seat while she rang the guy I'd spoken to the day before. After about five minutes, he came downstairs, shook my hand and asked me to follow him into this boardroom and told me to take a seat while he went to fetch his colleague. It was a real fancy room with a huge boardroom table in the middle, surrounded by leather chairs and I think his idea was to try and impress me with it but I couldn't have cared less. He came back in with this other guy and they had a look through the comic and were laughing at all the right places (Phew)

SECTION 1: HIGH

The other guy said that he would love to read it properly and thought there would definitely be a market for it on the internet. When I pointed out to them that the drawings were pretty basic and unprofessional, they both said that it didn't matter in the slightest.

"Look at South Park," said the other guy. "the drawings are very crude and yet it's massively popular"

They both said they liked the idea of people subscribing to it but didn't seem too interested in my idea of having people send me their comics, so I could make them look professional. (When I say me, I mean get someone who knew what they were actually doing to make them look professional)

I thought that was the best part of it but didn't say anything and went through with them about changing the name of Fireball to Darren Allen and when they found out he was a window cleaner, they both burst out laughing. Looking back now and it is so embarrassing. Of course he'd say they wanted my business and would have said anything to make me spend money with them. I explained that if it did work and become a success, then I wanted the real Darren Allen to have a 5% stake in the business. Anyway, the bottom line was I needed to raise £20,000 and I told them I would be in touch.

On my way back home, I was thinking about the website and how to advertise it and remembered seeing those tiny Smart Cars driving around with people's website addresses on them. That's what I needed to do, get one of those cars and get my address on it, of course! Arriving back at my flat at 4pm, I started to clear out my Galaxy of all the tools lumbering it up because I didn't need them anymore now that I was going to become an internet giant!

The Galaxy was a seven seater but I'd removed the back five seats so it acted more like a van and cleaned it inside and out before driving to my wife's house and getting the other seats out of the shed. Once they were all back in the vehicle, it actually looked pretty good and nobody would have known that it had been full up with timber and tools and I planned to drive to the nearest Mercedes/Smart Car garage first thing in the morning. When I got back home again, I opened the mail which I'd left on the table earlier and one of the letters was from a credit card company I had applied for. They had refused me and that brought my feelings down and made me pissed off, so I changed the wooden hand to a fist and went down the pub.

Apart from Josh serving I was the only customer (it was darts night and the witch's team were playing the pub furthest from my flat)

I wasn't in much of a talkative mood and my mind was racing with ideas of how to raise the £20,000 but each one came up a dead end. It got to about half ten and I was drowning my sorrows, when in walked Wendy the witch, Duncan the landlord, Tony the darts team captain and Bethany (Tony's daughter)

They all sat down at a table nearest to the bar where I was leaning and Bethany commented on how miserable I looked. I told her that I was okay but she kept on at me (she was a bit drunk) and so I told her that I had some problems and she wouldn't understand. With that, she stood up and started shouting, "Problems, problems. You don't know what fucking problems are!"

SECTION 1: HIGH

I started to shout back at her something about all the troubles I'd had as she called me an arsehole and stormed out the back for a cigarette. I was just about to follow her so I could carry on with the argument, when Duncan shouted at me to sit down.
"But she started having a go at me first and what problems can she have, she's only a bleedin' kid"
"I said sit down John; you don't know what you're talking about!"
Wendy looked at Tony who walked away to the other side of the bar and Josh came round through the hatch and whispered in my ear about Bethany and her past. This part is really difficult for me to write because it is of a very personal nature and although I've changed most of the names in this book, I still don't want to go into any details. All I'll say is that Tony walked away because he couldn't bear to hear any of what Josh was telling me about his daughter, the poor man. I was absolutely mortified at what I was told and felt so ashamed that I'd been shouting at Bethany and couldn't bear to face her when she walked back in, so I just walked out of the pub and made my way home.
About fifty paces from my flat and the drug dealer who'd been out the back of Wendy and Duncan's the other night, staggered up the road. He could hear me walking in his direction and looked up and shouted, "Alright Baldy!"
I've lost count the amount of times people have called me baldy and it doesn't bother me in the slightest, in fact it makes me laugh. Not because I find it amusing but it's the fact that these people can't think of anything funnier to say. It's a bit like in Cyrano De Bergerac where the guy calls him big nose and he comes back with all these witticisms, about twenty

times funnier and makes the man look such a fool. Anyway, this drug dealer had chosen the wrong time to take the piss and as he walked right up to me, I put the palm of my hand on his chest to stop him and said, "What did you just say?"

He started laughing in my face and said, "Alright bald…………….."

I picked him up and threw him into the middle of the road and then stood over him and slammed his head against the tarmac. I then grabbed him by the collar and raised my fist in the air.

His eyes looked manic and he'd obviously been on something. Spit was dribbling out of his mouth and he started laughing again.

"Fucking hit me…….. HIT ME!" he screamed.

I just laughed in his face and shoved his head back down on the road, "You're not fucking worth it, you prick," I said and walked to my front door.

He'd already seen where I lived before when he was walking past one night and so there was no point in trying to hide the fact. Once inside, I locked the front door and stuck a broomstick under the door knob and could hear him howling like a wild animal as he staggered up the street. Not knowing if he was going to come back with a load of his mates, I decided to stay up for a couple of hours and thought about what I'd do with all of my millions when I made it rich!

Thoughts began rushing through my mind at a ridiculous speed and so I got my notepad out and started writing down page after page of ideas for the website. Wide awake……..can't sleep! Full of energy. Why was I feeling like this? Fifty push ups to try and tire myself out but no use…….another fifty. I put some loud music on, not caring if Lydia was asleep next door.

"Those copyright guys loved my comic!" I said to myself. "The website is going to be huge and I'll be a millionaire in no time at all!"

My mind was racing out of control and the thoughts began getting faster and faster.

"The comic will be so successful that people will want to make it into a film and when that becomes a hit, I'll tell them that I want to direct a sequel!"

(Fucking bonkers!)

My eyes darted from one movie photo to another; they were everywhere, all around the living room. One to the other, one to the other, the next one, the next one, the next and the next and the next.

"I could make a brilliant film!" I thought. "I've seen so many, I remember so many. Every camera angle, every soundtrack. The way frames are lit, the dialogue, the characterisations. I know what's a good film and what's a bad one. It's not a matter of taste; films can be about any subject whatsoever. I might not like the subject but can appreciate whether it is good or bad!"

It was as if I were talking to someone else in my head but there was no one there.

"It must have a car chase in it and the actor must really be driving, like Steve McQueen in Bullitt. No CGI, no slow motion, no music!"

What the fuck did I know; I'd never studied film or even gone to college. To think I could direct a film without even learning about them was crazy.

It's like saying, "I work in a video shop, therefore I can make a movie!"

As if that could ever happen!

At the time, I just couldn't see that and in my mind I was already the next Sidney Lumet. I was driving myself mad!

"SHUT THE FUCK UP!" I screamed to myself and turned everything off and went upstairs.

Shutting the blinds, I pulled the curtains and closed the bathroom door because it had to be as dark as possible, without any street lights coming into the room. I got into bed, shut my eyes tight and the room was in total darkness but my mind was still racing with crazy ideas. Years earlier, I'd tried to quit smoking and bought an audio tape that teached people how to relax when trying to sleep. Remembering the instructions, I stretched my body out straight and starting with my feet and slowly working my way up, began to relax and become calm. It must have worked because…

CHAPTER 10

I woke up at 7am, washed and got dressed, climbed over my tools that were all over the floor after I'd cleared the car out and went over to Laura's for my scrambled eggs and smoked salmon. My arms and chest were aching and it took me a while to understand why, then I remembered it was from the push ups the previous night. When I got back, I knocked on the door of a fella a couple of flats down from me. He was a builder and had his own lock-up and I asked him if he could store all my tools for me and said he could use them whenever he wanted. He agreed and then I drove off to the Merc/Smart Car showroom to check out a second-hand motor. When I got there, I told the guy that I was looking for a used car about three years old and he pointed me in the direction of a load of cars, lined up outside. There were several that I really liked and noticing the salesman through the window, went back inside and saw a brand new black Brabus Smart car, gleaming under the spotlights of the showroom. It had these wide chunky wheels at the rear and an electric roof which folded right the way back, to turn it into a convertible. Looking inside I could see it had paddle shift gears on the steering column and smart, comfy leather seats and decided there and then, that I had to have it (even though it was more than three times the amount I'd intended to spend) and part-exchanged the Galaxy. They gave me the choice of three number plates and the last one on the list ended with the letters LSD (well, I had to didn't I)

A couple of days later, I went and picked it up and immediately drove to a car stereo shop, just down the road on the same industrial estate. The stereo already fitted in it was pretty standard and so I chose this Pioneer system with built in sat nav and a plug in the glove box to connect my iPod into. It had a touch operated screen and Bluetooth, which meant I could use my mobile phone hands free and look up numbers on the screen (state of the art at the time)

With the speakers and bass box in the boot and including the fitting, it came to £1700 (I just couldn't get rid of my money quick enough and by my money, I mean the credit card company's money)

I then took it to this other place and had the windows tinted and finally to another place and had the name of my website (which didn't even exist yet) put on the back window.

I must have told my sister Pauline about the car (she knew there was no way I could have afforded it) and she phoned me and told me to go and see my doctor. She'd been becoming increasingly concerned about me, probably due to the fact that I'd been ringing her and other members of my family in the middle of the night because I was wide awake and assumed they would be too. I can recall making all those phone calls but can't remember why and all I have to do is ask my family what I'd said but I'd rather not be reminded. Anyway, I promised that I would go see the doctor but didn't have a clue why she was worried about me.

After booking an appointment with the doctor for 2 o'clock, I went down the pub for a Guinness or two and Wendy was serving behind the bar and she asked me if I heard that wild animal screaming last night, just after I'd left. I played dumb and told her that I hadn't and had actually forgotten all about the drug dealer bloke and made a note to watch out for him. There was a guy named Richard sitting on his own in the pub, having a beer and reading a hunting magazine on his lunch break. He was a woodsman who looked after all the forest in the surrounding area and he'd split up with his wife quite recently too. I asked him how his day had been so far and he said that driving into work that morning, he saw a couple of cars pulled up on the side of the road and a group of people were standing in a field, next to a deer who had obviously been hit by one of the cars and was badly injured. He pulled over in his beat up old Land Rover and went over to the deer with a large knife and slit his throat. He said the people looked on in horror as he dragged it over to his car and managed to drape it across the bonnet and tie it down.

"That's my dinner sorted for the next couple of weeks!" he told me with a grin lacking most of his teeth.

The doctor seemed a nice enough bloke but must have only been in his early twenties and said my sister had contacted him and was worried about me because I was spending a lot of money. When he asked me if I was feeling anxious about anything, I told him that I missed my kids a lot but thought to myself, "He's only a kid himself, how can he understand what I'm going through? You can't read about these sorts of emotions, you have to the live them"

The doctor asked me if I had feelings of being superior and stronger than other people and I said no but there was a part of me that really did. Just saying, "I did" really over simplifies it though; it's not that I looked at

people and thought they were weaker than me, more that I'd discovered a way of having endless amounts of energy and they never knew my secret and how to get it themselves (without taking speed, that is)
Anyway, he diagnosed me with Bipolar Disorder which I'd never bleedin' heard of and gave me a prescription of drugs to take. I thanked him, took the prescription and went to the nearest chemist to get the meds. When I got back to the flat, I was just about to take one of the tablets when I suddenly changed my mind and threw them in the bin.
"What the fuck does he know?" I thought, "There's nothing wrong with me!"

CHAPTER 11

I started applying for as many credit cards as possible, in the hope of raising the funds to have my comic copyrighted and out of the two I already had, one was up to its limit and the other wasn't far off. The network coverage on my mobile phone in the village was terrible and any calls I made, kept cutting out. I rang the card company which I still had some credit on and asked if I could have an increase of a further £10,000 and considered trying for the full £20,000 but thought that might be pushing it a bit.

They told me to hold the line but as I was listening to the "on hold" music, the reception started to break up and then finally cut out all together. I called them again and was put on hold again. There was loads of interference and so I grabbed the credit card and went outside. Still, the line was really bad and I started to walk up the road, trying to improve the reception. About three minutes later, I was standing in the middle of the car park next to the library and finally had a clear line. Eventually, the guy came back on and asked me for my card number.

"Phew, thank fuck I brought it with me!" I thought.

"And can you give me the reference number on the last statement we sent you," he replied.

Shit, I'd left it in the flat.

"Hang on a minute mate," I said and started running back to the flat, explaining to him on the way, my predicament.

"Are you still there?" I called out while jumping over Darren's bucket, stuck in the middle of the pavement.
"I've been here ages," said Darren, busy cleaning a shop window.
"Hello? Hello? Are you still there?"
I could hear Darren behind me, calling out something but I ignored him.
"Yes, I'm still here," said the guy on the phone.
Great! I was back at the flat and the statement was on the table, where I'd left it. I span it around and read out the reference number. No reply.
"Hello? Hello? HELLO!"
Nothing.
"FUCK, SHIT, CUNT!"

My neighbour Lydia spent most of the evenings that week, round mine and we had a different Mike Leigh film on every night (she started to become a big fan)
I'd bought a new shirt and it needed ironing, so one morning when Lydia was in the laundry room at the end of our row of flats, I put it on a hanger and hooked it on her door handle and put a can of Stella on the ground.
Some guys were converting an old shop and the rooms above, into flats opposite and I went over and hid behind their skip and waited for Lydia to come out of the laundry room. Eventually, she walked back to her flat carrying a big bag of washing and went up to her front door. When she saw my shirt, I could see her mouth the words, "The cheeky fucker!" and took the shirt, put it on top of her bag of washing and went inside.
About ten seconds later, the door opened slightly and a hand came out and grabbed the can of Stella.

SECTION 1: HIGH

"Good girl," I said to myself, with a grin on my face. The girl living next to Lydia, worked in London and I didn't get to see her much, as she worked long hours but would occasionally say hello if I bumped into her when she got home from work. Her name was Kate and she was a bit of a yuppie type who seemed nice enough but never went out to any of the pubs in the village and didn't really know anyone there and kept herself to herself.

My mate Paul who I worked with from time to time (when I had work that is) came round one Saturday night with his wife Lou and we went for a curry in my favourite Indian restaurant next to me. Paul loves guitar music as well and we planned to go along to Wendy and Duncan's pub after the meal. Kate was in the restaurant with her friend and we got talking to them and I told her that it was going to be a good night down the pub. She said they didn't have any plans to go anywhere after their meal and would go along and meet us inside. They left before us and I told her we'd see them later. The curry was as fantastic as ever and Paul and Lou reckoned it was the best they had ever tasted. When we got to the pub, there was a really good atmosphere and Steve Forward was playing (look him up, he's fucking awesome!)
Kate and her friend were over in the corner and they asked us to join them. Both of them seemed quite drunk but were in high spirits and I went and bought a round of drinks for us all. We were sitting next to this long iron pole which supported part of the ceiling and Kate got up and started to swing round it, pole dancing style. When Steve started playing the next tune, Kate asked me to dance with her and we went up and stood

right in front of him and did a routine like John Travolta and Uma Thurman in Pulp Fiction. I was normally a pretty quiet sort of person but lately, my confidence had gone through the roof and everyone in the pub was cheering us on. When we got back to the table, Paul said, "Fucking hell John, what's got into you? You're like a different person!"

"I dunno?" I said and we both burst out laughing. Later on, I went to the bar to get some more drinks and Wendy said that her daughter Zoe had a friend who would really like me and would be down the pub next Saturday.

"I'll be here!" I replied.

Paul and Lou came back to mine for a few drinks and when they finally left, I stepped outside and knocked on Kate's door, feeling a bit horny and in the need of some female company. Kate let me in and her and the mate were both still drinking. She got me a glass of red wine and I went over to the mate, who was sprawled out on the sofa and started snogging her.

"Look at him, with his arse in the air," laughed Kate, "he's on heat!"

I can't remember much after that because I was pissed out of my head but they must have eventually slung me out because I woke up the next day, back in my own place.

Monday morning came around and I had another meeting with Alex, to discuss the website. He told me again that it would be much cheaper if I did all of the time consuming stuff like changing Fireball's name every time it was written down and so I went to see Josh down the pub and asked him if he could call the chef out from the kitchen. I explained to him that I

needed some work doing and the majority of it would involve altering the main character's name.
(How could I do it? I was far too busy thinking of some other ridiculous thing to do)
He agreed to help and said he would come round to my flat after he'd finished his shifts at the pub, to do the work. Because all of the wording in my comic was written by hand, I wrote the name Darren Allen (the window cleaner's name) and scanned it. The chef then had to paste it over the word Fireball every time it was written, which was a lot! I went down the pub that night and Josh wasn't behind the bar. Wendy served me and I asked where he was.
"His best friend was killed in a car crash last night and he's really upset. I've told him to take a couple of days off," she replied.
"What happened?"
"The police think a deer probably ran out in front of him and he swerved to avoid it and crashed into a tree"
His mate had been one of the guys driving like crazy to the nightclub that time and I knew that one day, one of them was going to get killed. He was only 21.
I got a cab to take me to the really cool club that night and while I was there, I asked one of the bouncers if they had any vacancies. He pointed to this other doorman who was in charge and he said that they worked for an independent company who leased out doormen to different nightclubs. I told him that I knew a guy who was a registered doorman and was looking for work. The bouncer gave me a phone number and told me I could give it to him, so the next morning I rang the cab driver who took me to Paddington and gave him the number but explained that if anything

did come from it, then it would probably be work in Essex and not his part of London. He said that he was prepared to travel and thanked me a lot. I got a phone call to do one day's work for a lady I'd done stuff for in the past and all she wanted doing was changing the handles on her kitchen units, so I told her I could do it the next day. While I was there, the cab driver rang me and sounded very excited.

"I got the job John, I got the job! Next time you need a lift to you know where, I'll take you for nothing!"

I told him that it was no big deal and wished him all the best and maybe I'd see him working in a nightclub some time soon.

Saturday night and I got down the pub at about 8:30. It was really busy and Wendy's daughter Zoe was sitting down at a table with a load of mates.

She shouted over at me to join them and introduced me to the friend who Wendy had spoken about. She was really attractive and we got on immediately. Her name was Beatrice but everyone called her Bee and she was only twenty four. Part of me thought she was a bit too young for me but she seemed very mature and I didn't feel my age (I was forty one at the time)

We all ended up getting pissed and danced all night long and when I went out the front for a cigarette, Bee came with me and we started kissing. Everyone was telling us to get a room and we eventually ended up back at my place, which became an eventful evening and Bee ended up staying the night. The next morning at seven and I was wide awake and up and about, so I went downstairs and played some music on the laptop while Bee was calling out for me to come back to bed.

SECTION 1: HIGH

Someone had mentioned to me that Wendy's husband Duncan was a mason and a thought came to me that he might know someone who could lend me the funds to get the comic copyrighted.

I took a cup of coffee up to Bee and she said, "How can you be so wide awake? We didn't get to sleep until about four!"

"I don't know," I answered, "for the last few weeks, I don't seem to need hardly any sleep and am full of energy"

"Then get back to bed and use some of that energy up in here," she replied.

"I've just got to go and see Duncan about something and when I get back, I'll fuck your brains out! I promise"

She gave out a sigh, turned on her side and pulled the duvet over her head. It's was now about 7:30 and I was knocking on the front door to Wendy and Duncan's pub. There was the sound of bolts being drawn back and then Duncan opened the door in his dressing gown, with his hair all messed up and looking half asleep.

"John? For fuck's sake! Do you know what time it is?"

"Sorry Duncan"

"Don't tell me, you've left your mobile phone here again?" (I was always doing that)

"No, no Duncan, it's not that. Can I come in and have a quick word?"

"It's half seven in the fucking morning!"

"I know mate, it won't take long I promise"

"I don't fucking believe this!" he said and stood to one side, to let me in.

We sat down at one of the tables near the bar and he started rubbing his eyes and yawned all the time.

"This better not take long, I'm bloody knackered and want to get back to bed!"

"Somebody told me you are a mason"

Duncan stopped yawning and just stared at me, not saying a word.

"Don't worry mate, I won't tell anyone"

"What's this about John?"

"I need to raise twenty thousand for a business idea but can't get the credit from anywhere"

"What's that got to do with me?"

"Well, I was thinking you might know a bank manager or someone and could put in a good word for me"

"I really don't know anyone in that line of business who could help you but there's this guy who would be able to lend you some money. I haven't got a clue what the interest would be though"

I got the feeling that he didn't want to tell me much, me not being a mason and all and I wished I'd never asked him because I felt that I'd put him in an awkward situation. He was basically telling me to go and get the money from a loan shark and even though my mind was in a manic state, I still had the sense not to go anywhere near someone like that. I was back to square one and thanked him for his time, apologising once again for waking him up. By this stage, I'd lost all concept of time and felt that if I was up and about and wide awake, then so should everyone else be. Walking back to the flat, I was wracking my brains trying to think of a way to come up with the money but couldn't come up with a single idea. When I opened the front door, I saw Bee's shoes lying on the floor by the sofa.

SECTION 1: HIGH

"Shit, I forgot all about her!" I thought.
Turning the laptop on, I put on some mood music, ripped off all my clothes and crawled up the stairs on my hands and knees, purring like a cat.
"About fucking time!" she called out.

CHAPTER 12

A few days later, a mate of mine called Bill came round to visit and I showed him around the flat. He really liked it but said that I would be better off buying a place, rather than renting. I had intended to do that eventually but now he had suggested it, the seed had been planted in my brain and I had to do it straight away! We went down the pub (where else?) and he told me that he was off to Thailand for three months. For the last twenty years, from December to February, he goes out there and does what you would expect a single bloke to do. Bill is a brickie and he works from March to November, seven days a week and I first got to know him when he built the extension on our house. My father-in-law had helped on the extension (that's an understatement) he was absolutely fantastic and worked so hard and was so knowledgeable and we found Bill in the Yellow Pages. He came round to see us while we were digging the footings and even though he hadn't been recommended to us by anyone, we both had the same feeling that he was the right man for the job. He was very matter of fact and seemed to know exactly what he was talking about and told us that we could drive around and see some of the work he had done in the area.

Anyway, we decided to use him and he was just as good as we'd hoped so we used him on future projects and recommended him to friends and family.

SECTION 1: HIGH

My father-in-law and I worked alongside Bill and that's when he mentioned going to Thailand every year. He told us that he had two apartments out there but rented them out and didn't use them himself.

Neither myself, my wife nor her dad had the nerve to ask the obvious as to what he did out there and we would always laugh amongst ourselves and say, "Well, does he or doesn't he?"

So back to the pub and Bill asked me if I would like to go out there and meet up with him. He said that he could arrange for a taxi to pick me up at the airport and take me to this hotel, where I could take the lift to the roof level and he'd be there with a load of ex-pats, sitting round a swimming pool and being waited on by a string of nubile young lovelies!

"It sounds really tempting Bill," I told him, "but I dunno if I can afford it"

(Although I had been spending money like it was going out of fashion, I felt I had to use what was left to go towards my master plan of getting the comic online)

"It won't cost you that much," he replied, "you can stay in the same hotel as me which will cost you £10 per night and the most you'll need to take out every evening is about £20"

"Wow, is that all?"

"Yeah. The hotel isn't much to right home about, it's just a place to sleep and for twenty quid a night, you'll be able to get about two or three girls. The only other money you'll need is for food and drink, which are dirt cheep and for lots and lots of Viagra!"

"How many women do you reckon you've been with since going out there?"

"About two thousand"

"FUCKING HELL!"
"Always keep your money in the hotel safe behind reception, not the room safe. If it does go missing, then you are covered on insurance. I told this German guy to do that and he said he didn't trust the hotels and so he carried all his money with him. On his second night there, he was walking along the beach and this girl came up to him and started to flirt with him and fondle his body. When he got to the next bar, he realised that she had taken all his money!"
"I'll definitely think about it Bill," I replied.
He got out a pen and started to write something down on the back of a beer mat.
"Here's my mobile number in Thailand," he said. "I'm out there for three months. If you do decide to come out, just give me a ring and I'll organise the hotel for you"
After another beer and plenty of stories from Bill, we said our goodbyes and I told him that I might see him out there.
Back at the flat and I started to think, "Do I really want that? It's not really my thing" but the thought of going away did appeal to me and if I ever did change my mind, I had Bill's number. Just one minute's walk away from my flat, work was just being completed on a block of four brand new apartments. On the ground level, there was a car park and then on the first floor, there was a one bedroom and a two bedroom flat. The top floor consisted of the same and the two bedroom flats had a balcony. I'd noticed them every time I walked past and a few days earlier, looked in the estate agents window to see what they were going for. Two of them were for sale (a one bedroom and a two bedroom) and the other two were available for rent. I

emailed a friend of mine called Ross, who lives in Massachusetts and asked him if I could come over and stay at his for a week. Although I've changed most people's names in this book, I've kept Ross's the same as I'm sure he'd love to see his name in print and wouldn't give a fuck anyway. He replied that he'd like to see me and so I had my schedule for the following day. Firstly, I would go to the travel agents and book a flight to Boston (Ross said he'd pick me up from the airport) and then I'd go to the estate agents and arrange for a viewing of one of the new flats down the road. With the frame of mind I was in, I didn't think about doing something, I either decided to do it or not to do it.

So the next morning, I went to the estate agents and asked if they had any flights going. They told me I was in the wrong building and if I wanted to go on holiday, then I should go to the travel agents down the road. When I got there, I inquired if the one bedroom flat was still for sale (only joking)
The travel agent told me that there wasn't anything available for about a week and I explained that I needed to go in the next couple of days. I felt that I had to fly out as soon as possible (don't ask me why) and they said they'd contact me if anything became up. Back at the estate agents and they arranged a viewing for me that afternoon. I got back to my flat and telephoned a mortgage broker that my wife and I had used several times. I explained my financial situation (dire) and he said that I should contact my wife to see if she was willing to use our house as collateral towards me getting a mortgage...... FUCK! I paced around the living room, thinking, thinking,

thinking.

"How can I raise the money to get my website idea off the ground? Once that is up and running, all my troubles will be over!"

I started thinking about the website again and how I could fine tune and improve it. Getting out my notebook (which if looked at now, contains the ramblings of a total fucking nutcase!) I began writing down more and more ideas. I started to get on a massive high and in my mind; the website was already a global phenomenon! It would only be a short matter of time and then I would be a millionaire. I could pay back the money I owed my sister and brother-in-law in Australia; they lent our family business all those years ago when we were in trouble. I could pay back the money I owed my mum and dad they'd lent me when I split up with my wife. I could pay off the mortgage on the house, so my wife and kids wouldn't have to worry and she wouldn't need to do the ironing service any more. I could give money to Great Ormond Street Hospital. I could buy a white 1970 Dodge Challenger like in the film Vanishing Point. I could buy back the villa in Portugal, my uncle once owned, so it was back in the family.

I could, I could, I could………..

So now in a great and positive state of mind, I went and viewed the one bedroom flat on the top floor.

The first thing that striked me was how well it was built and what a good size it was. To be honest, I knew I wanted it even before I stepped through the front door and as we were leaving, I asked the estate agent if I could look at the two bedroom as well. I thought I might as well, while I was there (big mistake)

SECTION 1: HIGH

For me, the best thing about the two bedroom flat was the balcony because I could stand out there and have a cigarette. I've never smoked indoors; I don't like the smell of stale smoke on everything. The balcony was linked by two doors; one from the living room and one from the master bedroom and the spare room could be for when my daughter came to stay. I thanked the estate agent for her time and went back to my own flat. My mind was racing at 100mph again and I immediately rang the estate agents and put an offer in for the two bedroom. I didn't even have any money for the one bedroom but knew somehow, that I'd figure a way of getting it. They said they would contact the developer, an architect whose office was just across the road from me and get back to me in the morning. Shit….. in the morning. I wanted to know straight away! Now that I knew the layout of the flats, I came up with a brilliant idea! I could buy the two bedroom and one bedroom flats on the top floor and knock them into one, it all made perfect sense! One of the spare bedrooms could be my office for my "brilliant" website business; one could be for my daughter and the other for me. I'd have a spare bathroom for guests and the kitchen / living room would become a massive space for entertaining!

That showed you the state of mind I was in and how spontaneously I had the urge to spend money I didn't even have. The day before, I told Bill that I couldn't afford to go on holiday and yet, less than 24 hours later, I was planning to fly to America and had put an offer on the flats.

The next morning, I got a call to say that the architect had accepted my offer and I decided to go over and pay him a visit (maybe I could cut out the middle man!) I'm cringing when I write this bit because it's so embarrassing but it's also funny, so who cares. I took my comic with me and knocked on the door to the architects and asked the receptionist if he was available. She asked me what it concerned and after I'd explained, she told me to take a seat and went upstairs to see if he was free. After a couple of minutes, she came back and said that I could go upstairs. I explained to him my idea of knocking two flats into one and pointed out where I thought it would be possible. He got out the drawings and agreed that the place I thought a doorway could go, was load bearing. Here's the embarrassing bit.

I showed him my comic and explained to him my website idea and told him that it was almost up and running. (If you could see the comic, you would realise why it's embarrassing. It's really not that good and just because someone down the pub loved it; I suddenly thought it was great!) He probably thought I was a total lunatic but listened to me waffling on. I'm actually starting to blush writing this because it's all coming back to me now and I realise how much of an idiot I must have looked. I remember now that I took the comic to the travel agents too and showed the bloke and he said, "It's very violent!" I also went to my uncle's London workplace and asked him his advice about advertising the website. OH, THE EMBARRASMENT OF IT ALL! ……still, never mind eh.

I then asked the architect if he would consider selling the other two flats as well. That way, I would own the whole building and could rent out the other two myself. He said that he hadn't thought about it but if

SECTION 1: HIGH

the offer was right, he would consider it. I didn't have a fucking penny to my name and now I wanted to buy the entire building! I said I'd see him later and I gave him some old chat but it's not like that on the TV when it's cool for cats, it's cool for ca, a, a, a, a, ats! (Sorry about that, went off on a bit of a tangent!)

I went down the pub that night, content in the fact that all my plans were coming into fruition and received a phone call from the travel agents the next morning to say they had a flight to Boston in two days time but it would cost £700. I only had £500 left on my card and decided that I'd better leave it for now. I didn't know it at the time but in three weeks, I would have absolutely no money left and the last thing on my mind would be trying to buy a flat.

CHAPTER 13

December 2008.
It was the first Saturday of the month and Zoe, her boyfriend, Bee and a load of mates invited me to go out with them to a club to celebrate Zoe's 21st birthday. With money being no object (I couldn't raise the twenty grand but as long as I had spending money, then everything was okay) I hired a stretch limo to take us from the pub to the nightclub. It was a really good night and they were doing three drinks for the price of one before eleven o'clock. Half past ten and the bar was ten people deep, trying to get in as many rounds as possible before it got to eleven and we managed to get enough drink to last us for the rest of the night and were all getting slowly drunk. I went outside to the smoking area and Zoe and Bee and two other girlfriends were out there, talking amongst themselves. Zoe asked me if I liked seeing two girls kissing and before I had a chance to answer, all four of them had their tongues down each other's throats.
"Can I join in?" I asked
"Sorry, ladies only," replied Zoe and then made me promise not to tell her boyfriend. I could have quite happily stood there all night long, watching them have their fun but eventually, we all went back inside. A strange thing happened to me about an hour later. We were all having a really good time but then I started to get paranoid about people watching me and told everyone that there was a man in the club who had threatened to kill me over a past dispute. It was an out

and out lie and I knew it was but I was beginning to convince myself it was true.

(By now I was realising the doctor had been right and there was definitely something wrong with me)

I wandered off on my own for about an hour and Bee finally found me on the dance floor of the downstairs part of the club. She asked if I was okay and I told her that I had to leave. We got the limo back to our village and I started to feel a lot better and invited Zoe and her boyfriend to come back to the flat with me and Bee. Zoe's boyfriend put loads of old school dance tunes on and we all danced round the living room until about three in the morning, drinking loads of red wine. Eventually, Zoe and her boyfriend left and Bee went upstairs. I found some great tunes on the laptop and turned the volume down, went upstairs, got undressed and climbed into bed next to Bee and kissed her on the lips. She was out cold and snoring quietly to herself.

"Shit!" I said to myself, then rolled over and went to sleep.

My birthday was coming up in a week's time so I decided to have a party at Wendy's pub. I started getting a playlist sorted out on the laptop and went to a printers to have a load of invites made up with Jimi Hendrix on the front.

Duncan said that I could use an amp he had to hook up my laptop to and also a pair of powerful speakers I could borrow. He had a function room upstairs and I set everything up to try it out and turned the volume up halfway. Wendy came marching in and told me to turn it down because all the customers were complaining downstairs. The village I lived in was in the middle of nowhere and some of the people I was inviting, lived up to fifty miles away. There was no way they were going to make it. I asked the printer to make up a banner with my website name on it and I was going to pin it to the wall on the night of the party. The village Christmas lights had been put up earlier in the day and when it started to get dark, the whole place had a magical feel to it. Duncan was a member of the town council and he knew Ronnie O'Sullivan and managed to get him to turn the lights on. All I had to do was open my front door and stick my head out and I could see him pulling the switch.

"Come on Ronnie!" yelled Duncan, "Let's count down from ten!"

"You do it Duncan, you do it," said Ronnie dryly.

There were stalls selling roasted horse chestnuts, a live band playing in the street and a small funfair in the library car park. I'd bought a real Christmas tree in the afternoon and my flat looked really festive and cosy. After I'd stuck my head out the door to see Ronnie switch on the lights, I went back inside to get dressed. Bee came round and said that she'd meet me down the pub when I was ready and when she left, I stuck on The Stones nice and loud. I got so into the music that an hour passed before I got down the pub and when I eventually arrived, Bee wasn't to be seen and so I asked Wendy where she was.

"She's gone to the funfair with Zoe and told me to let you know, to meet her there," she said. I noticed that Wendy and Duncan were all made up and I asked them where they were going.

"For a curry with a load of mates," replied Duncan, "why don't you join us?"

"I'm supposed to be going to a club with Bee but I don't half fancy a curry!"

SECTION 1: HIGH

"Then come along with us, she's with Zoe anyway, at the funfair!"
Wendy elbowed Duncan in the arm and whispered, "You heard what he said, he's going to a nightclub with Bee"
"Yeh but John said………."
"Go and find her John and get to that nightclub!"
"All right Wendy, keep your hair on, I'm going," I replied.
She gave me one of her evil witch looks and that was my cue to leave the pub. I found Zoe and Bee on the 'throw the hoop over a peg' stool and went over to join them.
"Won anything yet?" I asked.
"Where the fuck have you been?" said Zoe.
"Talking to your mum and dad. Here Bee, do you fancy going for a curry in a minute?"
"No she doesn't, we're supposed to be going to a club!" interrupted Zoe.
"What do you mean 'we'? I thought it was just me and Bee going out tonight"
"She got fed up waiting for you and is going out with me instead!"
"What's the matter Bee, you lost your voice or something?" I asked. I could tell she felt embarrassed and she shook her head.
"No," whispered Bee and threw a hoop over one of the pegs.
"Where's your boyfriend then Zoe; stood you up has he?" I said.
"No!" she snapped, "He's got to work tonight!"
I didn't have time for this shit. Just because she had no one to go out with, she thought she'd split me and Bee up for the night.

"Have a good time girls, I'm going for that curry," I said and walked off, pushing my way through the crowds of people. As I'm walking down the street to the Indian restaurant, two female coppers were heading towards me. When we got to about five feet apart, one of them said, "Excuse me sir"
"Now what?" I thought to myself.
"Can you tell me where you got that tee shirt?" she asked.
"What?" I replied. I was wearing a tee shirt with a picture of Dave Gilmour from Pink Floyd, on it.
"David Gilmour," she said. "He's the main fucking man!"
I started laughing and told her that was the first time I'd ever agreed with a copper.

When I got in the restaurant, Wendy and Colin were sitting at a long table with about twelve friends. They asked me to join them and made a space for me. When the waiter came over, I ordered a Cobra and a "phal with extra chillies!" The food arrived and I took a big spoonful of the phal and put it to my mouth and swallowed. It nearly blew my fucking head off and I took out the bottle of wine from the metal bucket filled with ice, next to me and took a big gulp of cold water. I like hot curries but that thing was lethal and I had to leave the rest. While everyone else enjoyed their meals, I ordered Cobra after Cobra and got slowly drunk. There was a couple on our table, sitting opposite me and the woman started rubbing her foot up and down my leg and smiling at me. She was pretty fit but I wasn't going to try anything on with the husband there and so I put down some money on the table and told Duncan that I was going back to the pub. When I got there, Bee and Zoe weren't around and so I got talking to Lydia from next door. I told her that I had some beer at home and she said that she had a bottle of wine in her fridge. When we got back to the flat, she said she wouldn't be long and went into her place while I stuck some music on the laptop. After Lydia returned, we started drinking copious amounts of booze and all of a sudden, we heard laughing and cheering coming from outside. I opened the front door and three of the waiters from the Indian restaurant were dancing in the street and calling out, "Hey John, great music, great music!"

They all lived in London but spent five nights of the week sleeping in one bedroom above the restaurant and would borrow DVD's off me to watch, after the Indian had shut. Lydia looked through the doorway and started laughing and we told them to have a good night and then went back inside. She woke up at five in the morning, kissed me and then went back to her own flat. We didn't want anyone knowing we were sleeping together as it was a small village and news travelled fast and the last thing I needed was her two sons finding out.

Friday came around and was the night of my party down the pub. It was really busy but nobody from my invitations had turned up apart from some people in the village who drank at The Chestnut and I was feeling a bit pissed off.

Darren was there, dressed in a lime green, pin striped suit which was about two sizes too small for him and he was dancing away happily by himself. He obviously hadn't got a decent pair of shoes because he was still wearing his steel toe capped boots but at least

he'd cleaned them for the occasion. There was a girl from Ukraine who worked behind the bar at weekends and she was fucking gorgeous. Jet black hair with almond eyes and long dark eye lashes which she used to flutter at me as a joke. She'd met an English guy who'd gone out there to find a wife and ended up marrying him but she wasn't happy with the relationship and wanted to separate. Usual story; wants to live in England but has to get married to some poor mug first so she can stay. She really enjoyed the songs playing on my laptop and Wendy asked her to dance with me. We stood in the middle of the floor and started dancing and then everyone else joined in; it was a really good atmosphere. Out of the corner of my eye, I noticed Lydia's eldest son Jay (who'd done some work for me) giving me a dirty look and I could tell he knew I was sleeping with his mum. The music was pumping out of the speakers and my mind was racing.
"He knows, he knows. What the fuck am I gonna do?" I tried to avoid him for the rest of the night and as the bell went for last orders, he walked over to me and just stared at me.
"Fuck it!" I thought, "If I don't do something quick, he's gonna deck me!"
"All right Jay, how you doing?" I asked.
He just nodded in silence.
"Look Jay, I like you and didn't mean to do anything to upset you"
"What?"
"When I slept with your mum, I didn't mean to upset you but she's a grown woman and separated from your dad"
"You slept with my mum?"

He didn't know anything about it, I was being paranoid again
"Oh fuck!" I thought, "Why didn't I keep my bleedin' mouth shut!"
I could see him start to shake with rage and so I tensed up and readied myself for him to come at me but instead, he turned around and marched back to his brother Daniel and some of their mates. I took a large gulp of beer and looked over in their direction. Jay whispered something in Daniel's ear and then went over to his mates and said something. They all looked over at me and I don't mind telling you, I was scared. The second bell went for last orders and Lydia walked in and went up to the bar.
"Shit!" I'm thinking, "This has just got a whole lot worse!"
She got her drink, spotted me and then saw Jay and Daniel and quickly smiled at me before going over to join them. I was dying for a cigarette but daren't leave the room in case I was followed outside. At least I was relatively safe with other people around me. Jay said something to his mum and then I looked down at his hands and he was clenching them into fists. He looked livid and for a second, I thought he was going to hit Lydia and I didn't know what to do. Daniel came storming over to me and put his face right up against mine.
"You fucking slept with my mum!" he said.
"Daniel, come back here!" called out Lydia.
He stared straight into my eyes and I got ready for him to swing a punch at me.
"Dan, come here a minute," called Jay and he turned around and walked back to his brother. Jay whispered something in his ear and then to his mates and they all

went outside the front door. More and more people were leaving and Lydia walked over to me.

"What did you go and tell him for, you fucking idiot? He wants to kill you!"

"I thought he knew," I replied.

"Of course he never fucking knew, he's stoned! He always looks that way when he's stoned!" she yelled and stormed outside.

About half an hour passed and there were only a few people left in the pub, having afters. I went up to the Ukrainian girl behind the bar and asked her to go outside to see if Jay and his brother were waiting out there.

"What you want to know that for?" she replied in her sexy Russian spy accent.

"Just do it, please"

She could obviously tell that I was serious and did as I asked and when she came back, she said, "There is no one there!"

I was thinking to myself, "Shit that means they are back at my flat, waiting for me to come home!" and so decided not to go back there for a while. I poked my head out the pub door and looked down the street. There was nobody in sight, so I walked over the road and hid behind the bus shelter and called a mini cab on my mobile. I smoked one fag after the other, waiting for the cab and when it turned up, I asked him to take me to a nightclub. No luck on the woman front but at least I was out the way of Lydia's two boys and their mates. It was 4am when I finally got home and there was no one in sight, so I rushed in and put the broomstick under the handle again and went up to bed. "Night John," I said to myself. "Happy fucking birthday!"

CHAPTER 14

I decided it was best to lie low for the next few days and didn't venture out of the flat unless it was absolutely necessary (to buy fags and booze and the odd spot of food)
My sister Pauline started ringing me more and more often, saying that everyone was worried about me and why didn't I go down to see them, for a few days. I thought that was a good idea as it would get me out the village for a while and hopefully, things would have cooled off when I got back. Ellie my middle sister, moved to Southbourne over twenty years earlier and then Pauline (my eldest sister) moved down to Hampshire about five years later, followed by my mum and dad who lived five minutes walk away. I had now totally maxed out on all my credit cards and didn't even have enough money to buy petrol to get down and see my family.

4:45am
Monday morning and I loaded the car up with my laptop, some clothes and my precious comic and drove to my friend's house, whom I'd worked for a few years back. At the time I had been at his company, I'd worked really hard as the manager there and his dad said they were pleased with me and I was going to get a pay rise. This was welcome news as my wife and I were struggling to keep up with the mortgage and an increase in salary would have been most welcome. I can remember it was a Friday afternoon and my

friend's dad came up to me and said that they had given me a ten pound a week pay rise. I couldn't believe it as I'd worked so hard for them and they'd even reached a target turnover figure because of my help. My mate came upstairs to the office and asked how I had got on with the rise. I told him that I was really disappointed and had to go because I was meant to do the deliveries for my wife's ironing service. Seven o'clock the next morning and I was having a very rare Saturday off work and was still in bed. The phone rang and it was my mate who said he was sitting outside and wanted to talk to me. We ended up driving all over London before getting back to a pub near me and he brought the subject of my pay rise up. I eventually got a better rise but right now, I was totally skint and thought I'd pay him a morning visit, just like he had done to me. It was about a quarter past five in the morning and I parked up outside his house and rang his mobile. He answered half asleep and I told him I was outside and needed to borrow some money.
"It's just gone five in the morning John," he yawned.
"Yeah I know, can I borrow some money?"
"Come in but be quiet, everyone is fast asleep"
We talked in his kitchen for a while and he was concerned about me but I told him that I was fine and not to worry. He gave me some money and told me to be careful and I said that I'd see him soon. Once I'd left, I drove to the nearest petrol station and filled the car up to the brim and got on the motorway. My car was promoted as being able to drive four hundred miles up to Scotland on a full tank of petrol if driven at reasonable speeds but I drove one hundred and thirty miles to Hampshire with the accelerator pedal

never leaving the floor and got there with just fumes left in the tank.

For the whole journey I stayed in the fast lane, constantly checking my rear view and wing mirrors for police cars and everyone was getting out of my way. It must have looked pretty funny with this tiny little car zooming past Porches and Mercs and I found that I really had to concentrate for the whole journey. I missed the Bournemouth junction on the M3 because I was thinking so hard about the driving and was heading towards Southampton and so rang my mum.

"John? Where are you?" boomed her voice through the stereo speakers.

Because of the speed I was doing and the car was a soft top and the engine was only inches away, the noise was deafening and so I had to shout to make myself heard.

"I'm on my way to yours!" I yelled, "But I've missed the turning for Bournemouth! How do I get back on it?"

"You shouldn't be speaking on the phone while you're driving!" she replied.

"It's hands free mum!"

"What?"

"It's hands free, I don't have to use my hands!"

I could tell that she'd covered the mouthpiece of her phone but could still hear her talking to my dad.

"He's not right," she said, "he's driving without using his hands"

"Tell him, he's got to use his hands!"

"John! You've got to use your hands, or you'll crash!"

"The phone mum! The phone is hands free!"

"How d'ya mean?"

"I don't have to use my hands to…….. hold up! Here's the turning, I know where I am now. See you soon mum!"
"John! John?"
"Gotta go!"
The last thing she must have heard was the screeching of tyres as I swerved to get to the exit just in time. Travelling at 70mph and without any traffic, you could get to my mum and dad's in about 2 hours, 10 minutes. I got there in an hour and a half and felt exhausted when I got out of the car. My mum and dad could see I wasn't right as soon as they opened the front door but I thought there wasn't anything wrong with me and sat in the kitchen with them, explaining my website idea.
"It's all been done already," said my dad.
"It hasn't," I replied, "if you look on the internet, there's nothing like it"
He didn't seem convinced and by the way I was ranting and raving, I don't blame him. Every so often, I would go outside for a cigarette and start to cry because I missed the kids so much and when I went back indoors, I'm pretty sure they knew I had been crying but didn't say anything. I went into their living room and got a photo of the kids off the top of the cabinet, sat down with it on my lap and tears just started to roll down my face. My mum came in and asked what was wrong and tried to hug me but I walked away and went outside for another cigarette. I didn't know why I had become so upset since being at my mum and dad's house, maybe it was because they reminded me of my children. The following morning and mum and dad went out to get some shopping. I rang the credit card company and this time, the

reception was good but the response wasn't. They declined an increase and so I rang my other card company. Same outcome. Shit! I spent the rest of the day sat at the kitchen table on the laptop, trying to find someone who would give me a loan

That evening, my sister Ellie rang me at mum and dad's and said she was at Pauline's and asked me to go round and see them.
"I'm knackered Ell, I might go to bed in a minute," I replied.
"Oh go on John," she said. "Bring your laptop. I've never seen your comic before"
"I'm really not in the mood"
"Please John; I haven't seen you for ages!"
"Oh……all right then. I'll be round in about half an hour"
Pauline lives five minutes round the corner and so instead of driving, I decided to walk. After putting the laptop in its case, I put on my coat and popped my head in the living room where my mum and dad were watching T.V.
"Won't be long, just going round to Pauline's for about an hour"
"Okay, see you soon"
When I arrived at my sister's, I noticed that Dave's car wasn't there, which I thought was strange as I hadn't seen him for a while and he was always such a sociable bloke.
"Must be working late," I thought to myself.
Dave is my brother-in-law and is the chef at a registered charity organisation which cares and houses people with learning difficulties.

He'd always told me I should go and visit because he said I'd love it but I just never found the time.
I knocked on the door and Ellie answered.
"All right Ell"
"Hi John, come in"

7pm, Tuesday 16th December
I went inside Pauline's house and was having a beer with my two sisters and asked Pauline where Dave was. She said he had to go out but would be back soon. Ellie asked me to set up the laptop, so she could look at the comic and as we were sitting on the sofa there was a knock on the door. Pauline got up to answer it and I heard a female voice I didn't recognise, talking to her. I looked at Ellie as if to say, "Who's that?" and she just shrugged her shoulders. All of a sudden, in walked three coppers, two men in suits and a middle-aged lady. I thought to myself, "eye eye, what's going on here?" and then immediately realised what was happening. The two men were psychiatrists and the woman was a social worker. One of the coppers stood by the front door, another in the doorway of the living room and the last one in front of me (I was still sitting down)
The shrinks sat on another sofa and the social worker sat next to me. I turned my head and looked up at Pauline and Ellie who were standing next to each other; neither of them saying anything. One of the psychiatrists asked me why I had been getting so tearful lately and turning back to look at him, I asked if he had kids or was he married. He didn't reply but instead, lifted his hand and showed me his wedding ring with a look on his face that said, "Of course I'm

married you idiot, what do you think I'm wearing this for?" (well, that's what I thought he meant at the time)
"That doesn't mean a thing," I told him. "you might be married but not have any kids"
He put his hand down and said nothing and then the social worker started talking to me in a really patronising tone.
"We're here to help you John, you're not well," she whispered and put her hand on my leg.
"Did I say you could touch me?"
She removed her hand and smiled. The second psychiatrist had been busy writing things down in a notepad and he looked up and said, "There's no need to lose your temper John, please keep calm"
"Do I look like I'm not calm?" I replied. "I very rarely lose my temper, doctor. In fact, I'd say I'm as cool as a cucumber"
"Is that why you hit that man in the street?"
"What man?" I replied and then remembered the incident with the drug dealer and mentioning to Pauline one time. I turned to look at her but she was staring down at the floor.
"I didn't hit him and anyway, that was one of those rare occasions"
"We know you're calm John," said the social worker. "We just want to talk to you"
"Well guess what……. I don't want to talk to you," and with that, I stood up and went to the living room door. The copper standing in the doorway looked at the two psychiatrists and one of them asked me, "Where are you going?"
"In the garden for a cigarette"
"That's okay," he replied and the policeman moved to one side, to let me through.

The copper, who had been standing directly in front of me, followed me outside to the garden and I lit up a cigarette and started cursing the shrinks and the social worker under my breath.
"They haven't got a fucking clue," whispered the policeman.
"What?"
"Those fucking psychiatrists. They think they know it all!"
"Yeah, you're right there," I replied, surprised by the way he was speaking to me.
"When I came out of the army," he continued, "I split up with my wife and couldn't see the kids any more and she got the fucking house!"
"What happened?"
"I just couldn't deal with being back in civilian life. This doctor told me he knew how I was feeling and what I was going through. How the fuck would he know?"
"What do you think they are going to do to me?" I asked him.
"I honestly don't know mate, we were told to attend in case you became aggressive. That's clearly not going to happen"
"There's no point, it wouldn't solve anything," I said, "it would only make things worse"
Just then, the wedding ring psychiatrist came outside and tried to have a conversation with me. I blanked him and talked to the copper but realised that he had all of a sudden, clammed up and didn't reply. After another cigarette, I went back into the living room and the social worker told me that I'd been placed under section 2 of the mental health act.
"Marvellous!" I thought to myself.

SECTION 1: HIGH

"We've tried to get you a bed in one of our Hampshire hospitals," she explained, "but unfortunately, there aren't any spaces and so you'll have to be admitted to a hospital close to where you live in Essex"

I looked up at the copper and he stared down at the floor and then I turned to my sisters. They both had tears in their eyes.

"Can I go back to my parents first, so I can get some more clothes?" I asked her.

"I'm afraid not, you have to leave straight away"

Getting to my feet, I walked over to my sisters and kissed them on the cheek.

"Don't worry, I'm okay," I whispered.

The three policemen took me out to a meat wagon and just as they were about to shut the door, the social worker walked up to me and said, "Everything will be fine John, it's for your own good"

"Fuck you, lady!"

SECTION 2: MEDIUM

(of the mental health act)

CHAPTER 15

The shrink hating copper started driving to the nearest police station, while I sat in the back of the van. I rang my cousin Lee on my mobile phone and explained the situation (he couldn't believe it!) and said that he would see me tomorrow. I then asked the copper if he could go round to Pauline's the next day and tell her I was okay (she was very upset)

He promised that on his way home from work tomorrow, he would go and see her (and he did too!)

We arrived at the local police station and thankfully I had a full pack of cigarettes on me because I needed them. I recall it being freezing cold because I was shivering as I smoked in the car park. You could tell that all three policemen didn't smoke, they looked really pissed off having to wait for me to finish my fag. I've forgotten the name of the copper who befriended me but all I can say is that he helped me a lot and I am very grateful to him. Inside the police station he got me a cup of coffee and we were chatting when another policeman walked in and said that I had to go with him. We walked back outside to the car park and I immediately lit up another fag. He explained that they were going to take me to another police station and would then drive me back to Essex and to the hospital. On the M27 on the way to the next police station, I realised that we were coming up to a service station and asked them to pull in as I needed to buy a bottle of coke (after the beer at Pauline's, I was really thirsty)

I remember these two coppers either side of me as we walked up to the kiosk and the look on the woman's face behind the glass. She must have thought I was either a detective or a convict and as she gave me my change, I winked at her. After what seemed like ages, we finally reached the other police station and after having a much needed piss and smoke, these two different coppers put me in the back of a van and locked the cage I was sat in. They apologised to me but said that I wasn't allowed to sit with them in the main part of the vehicle.

We drove all the way back to Essex and my arse was killing me because I was sitting on the rear wheel arch and I had to keep lifting myself up with my hands slightly because there wasn't enough room to stand up. I had to keep telling them to pull over as I needed a fag (ha ha)

We eventually arrived at the hospital at 11pm and these two coppers walked me into the reception area. I was tired and looking down at the floor and came upon these massive pair of shoes. Feeling physically drained I looked up and up and up into the eyes of this giant black man, who had such a kind and caring face. He must have been about six foot eight and I remember looking at these huge pair of hands as he gave the policeman a form to sign. Stretching up, I put my hand on his shoulder and said, "Ah mate, how you doing?"

He smiled down at me and took me through these set of locked doors and escorted me down this long bright corridor.

"Here mate, I'm dying for a cigarette!" I told him.

SECTION 2: MEDIUM

"You have to see a doctor first and fill out some forms and then I'll take you downstairs for a smoke before I show you to your bed" he replied in a strong African accent.

We came to another door and he pressed a button next to it. Through the glass panel, I saw this lady looking at me and then she must have pressed a door release button on the inside because there was a buzzing sound and the big guy opened the door and told me to go through. I walked into this large hall with round tables in the middle and some sofas at the far end. Immediately to my right was a glass box about twenty feet square and filled with light, which cast a glow over the unlit hall. The big fella told me to wait where I was and walked into the glass box, which I rightly assumed to be the nurse's station. He gave the nurse some paperwork and then showed me over to this other door on the left and told me to sit on the chair outside and wait for a moment. He went inside this other room and I heard him talking to another man through the door and then came out again and told me to go back in with him. There was this doctor sitting at a desk in a small room and he asked me to sit down.

"What is your name?" he said in a Polish accent.

"John Barrett"

"Date of birth?"

"Eleven, twelve, sixty six"

"Address?"

"Blah, blah, blah"

"Do you hear voices?"

"What?"

"Do you hear voices in your head?"

"Only yours Doc"

He rattled on for about another ten minutes and explained that I had been placed under section 2 of the mental health act, which meant that I could be held for a maximum of twenty eight days while I was being assessed and if I were deemed to be mentally ill and a danger to myself or to others, then I could be held indefinitely. The big fella walked back in and said that he'd show me to my bed and I quickly reminded him that he promised I could have a cigarette. We went back through the main door, turned left and down these concrete stairs and as we turned a corner, I noticed blood splattered on the wall. At the bottom of the steps was a small square area with two sets of double doors, opposite each other. We went through these glass doors to the left and were out in the open and he told me that I was now able to have a cigarette. While I smoked, he didn't say anything and just stared at me and so standing on the spot, I took a look at my surroundings. It was hard to see much in the dark but to my left was a high wire fence with barbed wire on top and in front of me, a steep grass slope with a flight of wooden steps running up to a level grassed area. It had turned really cold and the big man stamped his feet up and down and rubbed his hands together.

"Finished?" he asked.

"Let's go," I replied and flicked my fag against the grass slope. As we walked back upstairs, I asked him his name.

"Victor"

"Nice to meet you Victor, I'm John" I said and shook his hand which swallowed mine up.

"I know it's John"

"Oh yeh, right"

SECTION 2: MEDIUM

Back in the main hall and it was totally deserted. Victor told me to follow him and we walked to the far end of the hall, passed the sofas and turned right into a dark corridor. We passed a door and some windows on the right and came to another set. Victor opened the door and pointed to a bed in the middle of another two, which were hidden by curtains and the sound of snoring coming from behind each one.

"That's your bed John, in the middle. Have a good night's sleep and I'll see you in the morning," and with that, he turned around and walked out the door and shut it quietly behind him.

I sat on the end of the bed and peered around in the gloom. The room didn't consist of much, just a sink in the corner, two armchairs and a row of windows facing the outside of the building and so I got up and walked over to one of the windows and opened it. The gap was barely wide enough to get a hand through and down below, I could just make out a car park.

"I'm not going to sleep, I'm not going to sleep!" I told myself. "There's nothing wrong with me. I'm staying awake until I see a doctor first thing in the morning and get out of this place. I'm not going to sleep until I'm back in my own bed!"

I opened the door and walked back down the corridor to the hall. Peering round the corner, I could see Victor and the female nurse in the glass box and opposite, I spotted a vending machine. I quietly went over to the machine and got myself a cup of black coffee and sat down at one of the dining tables.

"I must stay awake. I'm NOT going to sleep!"

Victor looked through the glass of the nurse's station and noticed me sitting at the table. He got up and walked through the doorway and up to me.

"Go to bed John, it's late"
"No, I'm not tired. I want to sit here for a while"
He didn't reply and walked off down to the corridor I'd just come from. The nurse stuck her head round the door and asked, "Why are you not in bed?" also in a thick African accent.
"I just told Victor, I'm not tired"
She tutted and said, "Drink your coffee fast, then back to bed!"
"No!"
She tutted again and sat back down at her desk, shaking her head. I looked up at the ceiling and it was covered in paper chains and lanterns and over on the side was a Christmas tree with parcels around the base. Gold tinsel was stuck around the windows to the nurse's station and there were cards fixed to the edges of the glass. It was nice that someone had made the effort but it didn't put me in the festive mood one bit. Victor appeared from another corridor to my right and I guessed that the passageways must have gone round in a square shape. He looked over towards me as he went back to the nurse's station and said, "Bed" in a low voice.
I shook my head and went over to the windows behind me. Looking down, I could see a courtyard with a basketball court laid out on it and my guess had been right because the building went right around it, with high walls and windows on every side. I got myself another coffee and was dying for a cigarette but Victor had taken them off me when we came upstairs. Luckily, he had forgotten to see if I had anything else on me and my mobile phone was now hidden in my sock. I sat back down again and forced myself to stay awake. At about 4am, the female nurse did a tour of

the ward and didn't bother trying to persuade me to go to bed (I think they'd gotten the message)
When she went back into the nurse's station, I got my phone out and from under the table, sent a text to my cousin Lee, explaining where I was.
The Polish doctor had told me that I was due to see another doctor at 11am and so I spent the rest of the night thinking how I was going to talk my way out of this situation.

CHAPTER 16

7am, 17th December.

All of these patients started wandering into the hall like zombies and from out of the corner of my eye there was this one woman who must have been 6, 3" with wild eyes and hair all over the place. She continuously made this low groaning noise and she scared the shit out of me. I was dressed quite smart and all of these people kept coming up to me and asking if I was a doctor. I said no and so they asked if I was a patient and I replied, "Definitely not!"
More and more people started piling into the hall and I kept my gaze on the table top, so as not to stare at them
"I'm not one of THEM!" I thought to myself.
I was aware of someone standing over me and then sitting down on the chair, to my left. This woman placed her hand gently on my arm and asked if I was okay and without looking up, I told her to leave me alone. She said she was an advocate and had been a former patient herself and knew what I was going through. I looked at her and could see she was genuine and so I started to tell her about myself and how I ended up in this place. I was rattling on and on, talking about missing my kids and when I looked up at her, she had tears in her eyes.
"I'm sorry," she said. "I know I shouldn't do that but when I hear so many sad stories, it really upsets me"

SECTION 2: MEDIUM

Her colleague came over and said that they would attend the meeting with the psychiatrist and speak up for me on my behalf.

"What's the chances I can be out of here today?" I asked.

They looked at each other and the colleague said, "We'll have to see how it goes when we see the doctor. If you feel you want to speak up for yourself, then by all means do but remember we deal with this kind of thing all the time and know the right things to say"

I looked around the hall at all of the patients and they all seemed to be staring at me. Victor went downstairs with me, so I could have a much needed cigarette and I got to see my surroundings in the daylight. The wire fence turned out to be a secured enclosure with more patients inside and one of them pressed his face against the metal and asked me for a cigarette. I explained to him that Victor had my cigarettes upstairs and the one I was smoking was the only one I had on me, so he looked at Victor and asked him if that was true. Victor nodded and then told me that we had to go back upstairs and as we walked away, I passed the rest of my cigarette through the wire mesh, to the guy on the other side. When we got back to the main hall, most of the patients were sitting down eating breakfast and Victor asked if I wanted any.

"I just want to see the doctor and get out of here," I replied.

10am and my cousin Lee arrived. We went into what I later found out to be the quiet room and he looked at me and we both started laughing but in a nervous kind of way. He had a carrier bag with him and from it, he produced a bar of chocolate, two packs of fags, a lighter and a 'gentleman's magazine'

"That's the last thing I need at the moment!" I joked.

"Oh I don't bleedin' know, give it to one of the nutters and they can bang one out in front of the nurses!" he replied.

I told him to wait there a moment and went to my room and stashed one of the packets of cigarettes and the lighter under my wardrobe. When I got back, he said, "How'd ya end up in here you silly sod?"

"My family set me up; they think there's something wrong with me"

"You seem the same to me, as stupid as ever!"

"I've got to see the doctor in twenty minutes. Will you come in with me?"

"Yeh, of course boy"

The advocate, who seemed to be in charge, came into the quiet room and asked if I wanted to go for a quick cigarette before going in to see the doctor.

As we passed the nurse's station, I told her and Lee to hold on and handed over the other pack of fags to Victor who wrote my name on them and put them with the other patient's cigarettes. Outside, Lee said, "What d'ya give him your fags for, you mug?"

"I don't want them thinking I've got any hidden and so I'm pretending to do everything by the book"

The advocate's name was Melanie and I felt so comfortable with her. Once we were outside, she backed up against the wall and lit up a cigarette and pointed to a camera above her head.

"This is a blind spot," she said, "they don't like me smoking in front of patients"

SECTION 2: MEDIUM

I eventually got to see the doctor, joined by Melanie and Lee. Victor was present and he handed some paperwork over to the psychiatrist and by this stage, I'd been awake for over thirty hours and was completely knackered.

Melanie began talking on my behalf and I respectfully told her that I'd like to speak for myself. I figured that this psychiatrist must hear the same thing all of the time from a patient's advocate and I wanted him to know that I was calm and had my wits about me. Once again, I was asked if I could hear voices in my head (it must be a common thing, I thought) and once again, I replied, "No"

"Your sister tells us that you've been driving erratically and in a dangerous manner. She is very worried about you," he said.

"I was only doing 80mph," I lied and tapped my foot against Lee's.

"I'm a very sensible driver," I continued.

Lee coughed and put on his most serious voice.

"John is a very careful driver and is probably the most sensible I know....apart from me!" he said and gave a nervous laugh.

The doctor smiled and whispered something to Victor. I was half asleep and Lee said, "Look, he's been awake for a day and a half. Can't you do this later, and I don't think he should have to share a room with other people. John's told me there are single bedrooms along the hall; he's bleedin' knackered. Now get this man a bed!"

The doctor whispered to Victor again and then said that they were full to capacity, so I'd have to stay where I was for the moment but they'd look into moving me when possible.

"When can I leave?" I managed to say, almost dropping off.
"By law, you have to stay here for at least three days while we assess you but if deemed necessary, we can keep you here as a patient for up to twenty eight days"
"And what happens after the twenty eight days?" I asked.
"If we feel that you have not improved or may still be a danger to yourself, we can still keep you here for observation"
"How long for?"
"Until we feel you are ready to leave"
I must admit that when I heard him say that, I was starting to get worried.
After my meeting with the doctor was over, I went downstairs with Lee and Melanie for another cigarette. She said that I had spoken very well and as soon as she heard anything, she'd let me know. Lee said that he had to get back to work but would come back soon and gave me a score.
Such a diamond geezer, he lives in Kent and works for himself and came all that way on a work day without a second thought. As he left, we hugged and I tried not to cry.

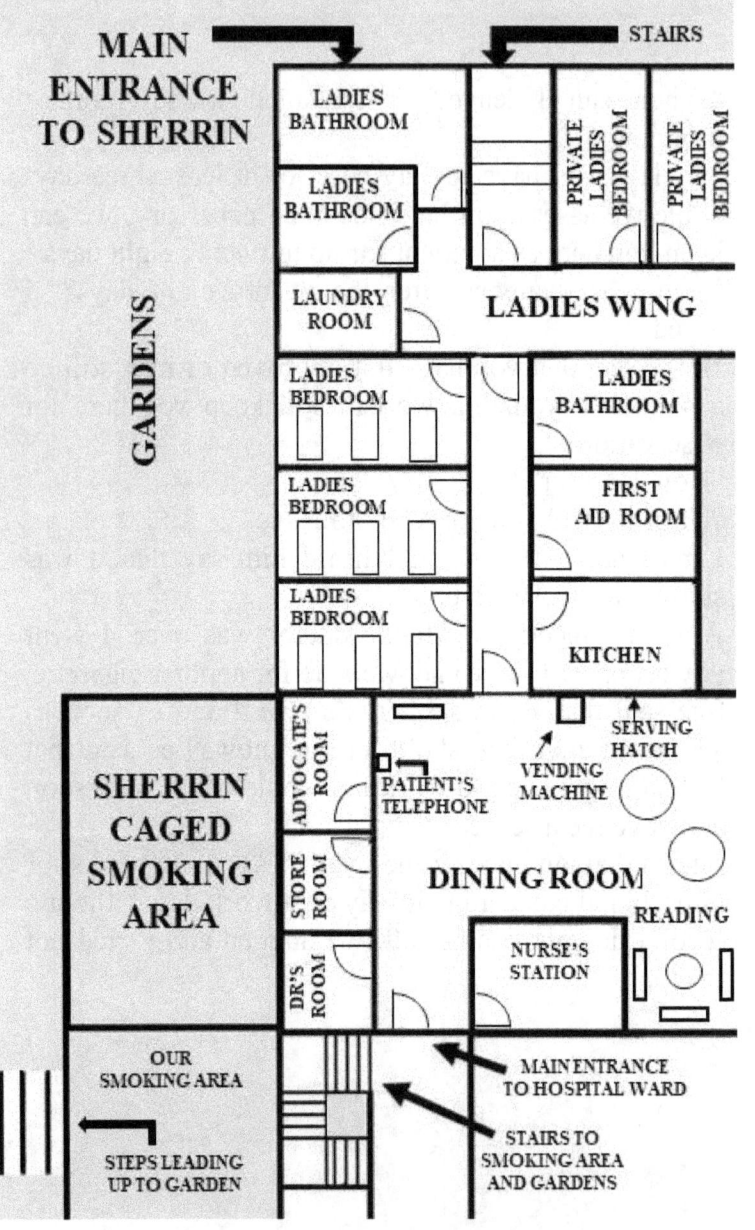

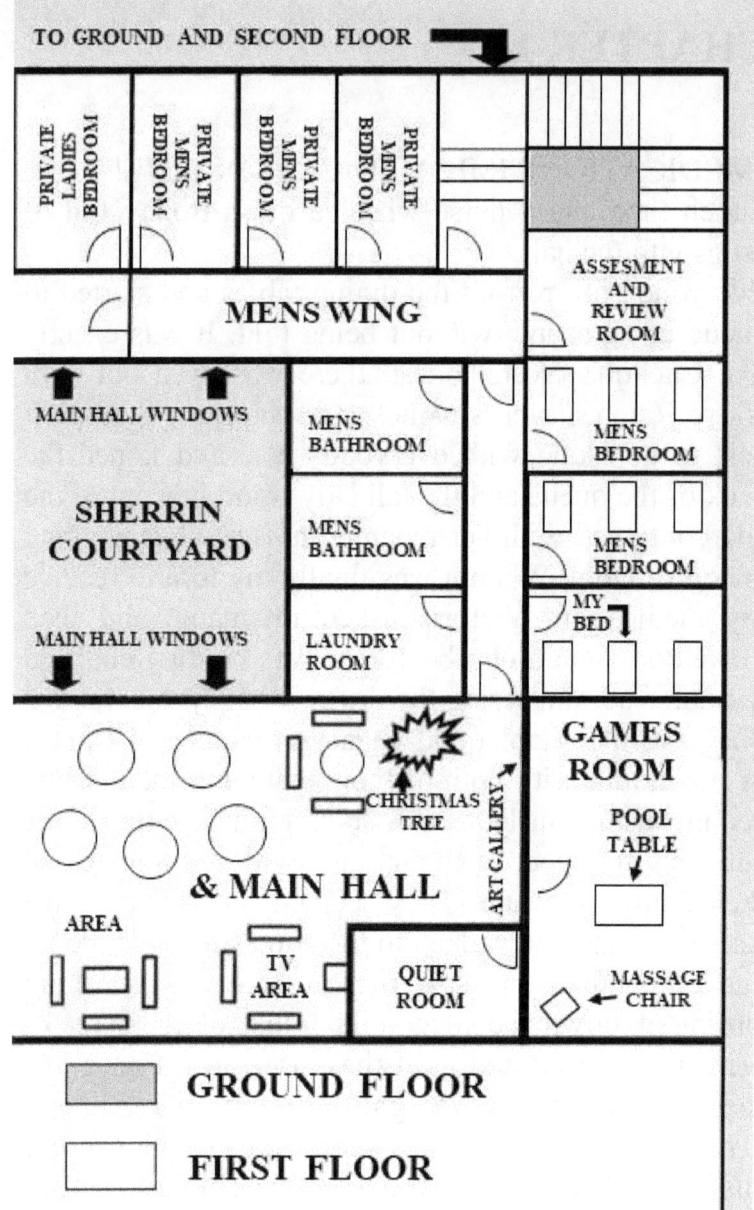

CHAPTER 17

"MEDICATION TIME, MEDICATION TIME!"
Lunch time and a nurse wheeled out a trolley full of drugs into the hall.
Everyone got up from the dining tables and started to queue up in a line, without being told. It was exactly like Cuckoo's Nest; honest, there was even our own Nurse Ratched who's name was Victoria. I thought it best to go along with everybody else and joined the back of the queue and the tall lady stood in front of me and continued with her moaning noises while shaking uncontrollably. When it was finally my turn to receive my medication, Victoria asked my name and then looked down at a clip board she was holding and told the nurse administering the drugs, what type I was on. She gave me a tablet and a glass of water and I put it in my mouth with both of them watching me closely. As inconspicuously as possible, I pushed the tablet between my upper teeth and gum with my tongue and then drank the water. They seemed satisfied and so I turned around and walked to the games room at the far end of the hall and spat the pill into a sink before rinsing it down the plug hole. Most of the patients were walking around as if they were in a trance and there was no way I was going to end up like them! Over the next two days, Victoria must have become suspicious because they changed my tablet to one that dissolved quickly in the mouth and so as soon as I'd drank the glass of water, I would have to get to the sink as fast as possible. Either that or another patient

would take it out of my mouth and have it for themselves. I witnessed loads of patients losing their temper with members of staff and realised that it was much better to stay calm.

The two other men in my room were complete opposites. The guy to my right seemed to do nothing but sleep and snore all day (loudly!) and to my left was a man called Zee. I can remember the first time I met him was when he walked into our room while I was sitting on my bed, eating the chocolate Lee had given me. There was a suitcase by one of the chairs and as soon as he saw me, he rushed over to it, opened the top and checked the contents.
"That's my bed over there and everything around it belongs to me!" he growled in a deep threatening voice.
Straight away I realised that the best thing to do would be to stay on his good side and so I offered him some of the chocolate and told him that I didn't want to touch his stuff. That seemed to do the trick and he came over, shoved the rest of the chocolate into his mouth, sat on the end of my bed and introduced himself (with his mouth still full)
We shook hands and I told him my name. The bag containing the porno mag was on top of my bedside cabinet and so I took it out and said he could have it.
"Nice one!" he mumbled, still munching on the chocolate.
I wanted to be safe in the knowledge that I could sleep soundly at night and not have the bloke next to me, getting up and strangling me or something. By giving him the magazine, I figured he knew I wouldn't steal his stuff. Zee had this look in his eyes which told me

he could snap at any minute and the last thing I needed was to be in his bad books. He was about six foot tall, with short cropped dark hair, an olive complexion to his skin and glasses that looked like they'd been bought in the early eighties. If you walked past him in the street you wouldn't have given him a second glance but if he came up to you and spoke, you would know not to mess with him. He was stocky without being overweight and always had this intense stare which could be quite unnerving. I looked at his hands which were always clenched into fists and noticed that his knuckles were covered in scars.

"I'm going outside for a fag," I told him, "do you want one?"

We got on really well and he told me all about himself, as I did to him.

There was this lady patient called Lucy who would go outside for a smoke every hour, on the dot. She was only little and I'm guessing, in her mid to late thirties with short black hair and had a really cheeky expression when she smiled (think of Malcolm McDowell's crooked grin in A Clockwork Orange and you've got it!) It was Lucy who'd asked me if I was a doctor on the first morning of my admission. We became great friends and after everyone else had gone to bed in the evening, we would stay up all night talking on the sofas by the television in the main hall. I would tell her all about myself and how I ended up in the hospital and she'd explain to me why she ended up there too but I felt she was keeping something to herself. Every so often, we would go to our rooms, sneak a quick fag by blowing the smoke out of the windows which only opened a few inches and then come back to talk some more. The nurses kept telling us to go to bed when they found us talking but we just ignored them. Lucy told me one night, that she had been raped by a cab driver when she was a schoolgirl and he'd taken her home from school and offered to carry her bags to the front door. As soon as she unlocked it, he pushed her inside and attacked her. I looked at her arms and they where covered in scars, where she had self-harmed over the years and staring into Lucy's eyes, you could see so much pain and suffering and yet on the whole, she was such a happy and friendly person.

She told me that she'd been admitted into this ward, about eight months ago and had tried to stab a female nurse with a dinner knife, one evening.

When I asked her why, she just shrugged and said, "I don't know"

I used to call her Steve McQueen because she was always trying to escape!

Whenever it was time for her cigarette, Lucy would shuffle over to the nurse's station, hunched over with her arms crossed and wait by the main exit for someone to take her downstairs. When no one was looking, she'd make a dash for the door release button and a member of staff would quickly rush out of the room and stop her and every time they did this, they would threaten her by saying she would go back into Sherrin. She'd been back in this particular ward for only a couple of weeks and had been transferred from Sherrin ward, downstairs. Sherrin was where they kept all the seriously dangerous patients (either to themselves or to others) and when I would go outside for a fag, you could see them in the giant cage.

SECTION 2: MEDIUM

On the rare occasions I did actually go to bed, I could hear the patients in Sherrin, directly below me. They would either be crying out in fear and anguish, or screaming with rage. The last thing I wanted was for Lucy to end up back there again and so whenever she made a dash for the door release button, I would quickly pull her away before any staff noticed.

"Don't touch me," she'd whisper and I would gently take my hands off her arms.

Eleven o'clock on the dot and everyone who smoked was queuing outside the nurse's station, waiting for someone to take us downstairs. I'm sure they would purposely make us wait longer than they had to and when we all finally marched down the steps and into the courtyard, we'd smoke as many as possible before the nurse would tell us to go back to the ward. On this occasion, I was standing close to the wire fence which surrounded the courtyard to Sherrin ward and a group of their patients came outside for a smoke too. One of them asked me for a light and stuck the cigarette through the wire mesh.

"Cheers mate," he said, "I ain't seen you before"

"I only got here two days ago"

While we were talking, I looked over his shoulder and noticed these two huge orderlies watching us. Without turning round, the guy said, "Yeh, I know, we're being watched. They're checking you don't pass something to me"

"Like what?"

"Anything but mainly a weapon. You got any kids?"

The sudden change of subject, threw me for a moment.

"Yeh, three. Two boys and a girl. You?"

"A boy and a girl. I used to give them their baths every night"
He started saying that it was ok to touch your own kids while bathing them and I immediately stepped away in shock. You just don't know about someone until you really get to know them and even then, you don't fully know what they are thinking. He seemed like a nice enough bloke to me and then he comes out with something like that. I asked Zee, who happened to be outside smoking at the same time, if the man meant what I thought he did and he said yes. Zee stared through the wire fence, straight into the eyes of this guy and I could see the look of rage on his face. The other man looked to the ground, stubbed out his cigarette and walked back into the building.
"Fucking cunt!" growled Zee, "I'll get him one of these days!"
Lucy was stood as far away from the fence as possible and was lighting up another cigarette.
"You all right Lucy?" asked Zee.
She nodded and took a deep drag on the cigarette.
"It's okay, he's gone now," he said.
Zee had been in Sherrin previously and knew just about everyone. He was a bit of a psycho but as I said before, we got on just fine. He didn't give a fuck and would just walk out and go down to the shops whenever he felt like it.
"What can they do?" he'd say to me, "nothing. Just bring me back here again!"
I'd give him money for booze and fags and he would stash them in one of the courtyard bins for me from time to time.
At about three in the afternoon, I was in the hall getting a coffee from the vending machine, when this

man walked in with Victor. They were both chatting to one another in a friendly manner and it would have been easy to assume that the other man was also a member of staff, except for the way he was dressed. He was very slim, probably in his early thirties and wore a ripped tee shirt and jeans. As he walked passed the nurse's station, he popped his head in and said hello to everyone and they all seemed to know him and waved back. I took my coffee and sat down on the sofa nearest to the exit, seeing if I could figure out who he was while Zee walked through the hall, making his way to the exit. He saw Victor and said, "Just going to get some fags from the petrol station"

"You'll have to wait until one of us is free and we can accompany you," replied Victor.

"Hello mate!" called the new man to Zee, "you still here?"

"Oi you old bastard, how you doing?"

The new guy walked over to Zee and shook his hand and I noticed him pass Zee a tenner.

"Usual?" whispered Zee.

"Yep"

"Won't be long Vic," called out Zee as he pressed the door release button.

"Come back here and wait for one of us"

"See you in a minute," replied Zee and he walked out of the ward. I looked at Victor through the nurse's station window and noticed that he made no attempt to go after Zee. The new guy looked around the hall and then down at me sitting on the sofa and walked over.

"My name's John," he said and held out his hand. If he's a friend of Zee's, then he must be okay, I thought to myself.

I shook his hand and replied, "Good name"

He sat down next to me and explained how he knew everyone.

"This is my fourth time here," he said and I noticed that he couldn't stop sniffing his nose. I wanted to learn more about him and decided it was only fair to tell him about myself too.

"You got your own room?" he asked.

"Nah, my bed's next to Zee's"

With that, he burst out laughing and replied, "He's a good guy Zee; just don't get on his wrong side"

"Why are you here?" I asked, "It's as if you've come of your own free will"

"I have….sort of. Roughly every six months, I feel the need to re-admit myself"

It turned out that John was a DJ and played at all the big clubs in Ibiza. Every so often, the hedonistic lifestyle became too much for him and he'd use the hospital as a kind of re-hab clinic.

"The first time, I'd just got back from San Antonio and was driving along when I had a panic attack and crashed the car. I didn't know what the fuck was wrong with me and my girlfriend got me admitted here," he explained.

"But what about all the other times?" I asked, "You can't just walk in off the streets"

"I go and see my doctor and tell him that I think I'm having a relapse. He's told me that I should change my job but it's all I know"

"So how long are you expecting to be here this time?"

"Only three days, it's all I need"

"How do you know they'll discharge you after only three days?"

"That's the minimum time they can hold you. They know the score; I'll be out in three days"

SECTION 2: MEDIUM

"Do you think I could be out in three days?" I asked.
"That depends"
"On what?"
"If you can convince them that you are in a fit state to be discharged"
"You must be on good money," I said, "why don't you go private?"
"The money's okay I suppose. The main problem is I spend it all on Charlie, besides……..I like it here. It brings me back down to earth"
"You like it here?" I replied in amazement, "How can anyone like it here?"
"How long you been here?" he asked.
"This is my second day"
"Wait until you've been here a bit longer, you'll understand"
"Never!"

I looked at John and he didn't reply and just smiled. To me, there was absolutely nothing wrong with John, he certainly didn't appear to be mentally ill and I really liked him. He reminded me a lot of myself and I could see how easy it would be to fall into his kind of lifestyle. John could have so easily have been an obnoxious person who bragged on about doing this and that (I've met a few of them) but he was exactly the opposite. He only said something when it needed to be said, just my type of person. When Zee came back, we went downstairs for a cigarette. He could see that me and John were getting on well and said, "I'm going to play some pool, I'll see you two later"

I'm not sure why he left us, maybe he could see that me and John had something in common that he didn't. Maybe he felt it would do me good to speak to someone else, I don't know. For the rest of the day, we talked and talked and when it came to the evening, I was really surprised he didn't join me and Lucy for our night time chat.

"I wonder where John is?" I asked her.

"He takes his meds, unlike you and is probably zonked out in bed," she answered.

"Do you take your meds, Luce?"

"Sometimes, I haven't been for the last couple of days"

"Why?"

"I'd miss our evening discussions!" she said and smirked that smirk of hers.

On my third day, I had another meeting with the doctor and somehow I must have convinced him there was nothing wrong with me because I was discharged on the Friday at midday. While I was waiting to be picked up, I went downstairs for a cigarette, accompanied by a female nurse and John appeared from out of the building.

"Where have you been?" he asked, "I've been looking everywhere for you"

"I've just had my assessment with the shrink, I've been discharged"

"You must have done something right then!" he laughed and shook my hand, "Take care mate"

"I'll miss you John," I said and tears started to form in my eyes.

He squeezed my hand and replied, "No offence mate but I don't ever want to meet you in here again"

I laughed, patted him on the shoulder and told the nurse I was ready to go back inside. As we were walking back up the stairs I said to her, "Don't tell the doctor you saw me upset"

SECTION 2: MEDIUM

I thought that if he knew, he might change his mind about discharging me. It sounds really silly now, why would he? Back upstairs I went to my room and said goodbye to Zee. He gave me a great big hug which nearly crushed the life out of me and I gave him a packet of cigarettes. I would have said goodbye to the bloke sleeping on the other side of me but he was still snoring his head off! I collected the few things I had with me and put them in a carrier bag and went out into the main hall. Lucy was standing by the vending machine and I walked over to her.
"I'm going now, Luce"
She looked up at me and said, "Going where?"
"Home, I've been discharged"
Lucy turned away from me and whispered, "I'll really miss you John"
"I'll miss you too mate," I said and put my hand on her shoulder. She quickly moved away from me and started to walk towards the lady's wing.
"Bye John," she said and disappeared from view, without turning around.

CHAPTER 18

Lee came to collect me and took me back to my flat (my car was still at my mum and dad's place in Hampshire) I quickly took a shower, had a change of clothes and then Lee drove back to his house, where I spent the night. His wife Sam was so nice to me and very sympathetic and I'd just like to take this opportunity to thank them both very much for all they did for me. The following morning, Lee drove me to my mum and dad's (never once asking for petrol money or anything like that)

When we arrived, I knocked on the door and my dad answered. He tried talking with me and said that I wasn't well but I completely ignored him and called out to my mum, "Have you got my car keys?"

When she came to the door, she looked upset but said nothing and handed over the keys. My dad went over to Lee sitting in his car and tried to convince him that I was ill. It must have been really awkward for Lee and I don't know what he said to my dad but he called out to me, "Shall we go John?"

I got in my car and pulled out of the drive, with Lee following behind in his own car.

When we got on the motorway, Lee shot past me and waved goodbye as he went past. I decided to keep to 70mph, all the way home (the last thing I needed was to get done for speeding!)

Back in my flat and for the first time in four days, I was on my own, not taking my medication and my

SECTION 2: MEDIUM

mind was still buzzing at 100 miles an hour!

I went down pub that night.

They had a different guitarist every Saturday night and this particular guy was great! His playing style and demeanour seemed to be influenced by Keith Richards. A Scottish bloke, who you wouldn't fuck with (6, 5" and smothered in tatts) got up on stage and started playing the harmonica with him (brill!)

I'd become friends with him and his girlfriend (who you wouldn't fuck with either and was also smothered in tatts)

I told her what had happened to me and when Al (her boyfriend) came off stage, she told him too. He said that he had been sectioned in Scotland and she had literally saved his life and as he was speaking to me, I noticed she was squeezing his hand in a reassuring manner. During the guitarist's interval, he went out the back for a cigarette and Al, his girlfriend and I joined him. The drug dealer, who I'd thrown into the middle of the road, was there with some mates. He was pissed and being a right prick, hurling abuse at everyone. Al and the guitarist were talking to each other and the drug dealer started to say, "Hey Jimmy, you all right there Jimmy. Och aye the noo Jimmy!"

I looked over at Al who was staring at the ground and I could see he was trying to control his anger. His girlfriend put her hand on his shoulder, whilst the drug dealer's mates burst out laughing.

"Oi prick!" I called out. "You don't remember me, do you?"

All his friends stopped laughing and were now staring at me, while he had a look of faint recognition on his face.

"Yeah, that's right prick; I'm the bloke who was this far away from caving your head in!"
One of his mates started to say something and I cut him short.
"I ain't talking to you; I'm talking to your wanker of a mate!"
"While I'm drinking in this pub, I don't want scum like you filling up the place. Now fuck off!"
He looked at his mates and then they all looked at me and Al and the guitarist and then they left.
After the pub closed, me and the guitarist went back to Al and his girlfriend's flat and Al opened the front door and told me to go in first. As I walked in, he shut the door behind me so I was on my own and I could hear him laughing outside. I was at the end of a long corridor and could hear a low grumbling sound coming from the far end. Suddenly, this huge fucking thing (which turned out to be an Argentinean hunting dog which I think is banned in this country) poked its head round the corner at the end of the corridor and saw me on my own. As you can imagine, I thought to myself, "OH SHIT!"
He came flying at me and there was nowhere I could go so I thought, "There's nothing I can do, who gives a fuck!"
I stood there with my arms by my sides and showed no emotion whatsoever. The dog jumped up at me, put his paws on both my shoulders and barked his head off with his teeth about six inches from my face! I just stared into his eyes and showed no fear whatsoever and just like that, he dropped to the floor and started whimpering. Al was outside, pissing himself with laughter and when he finally came in, he slapped me

on the back and said, "Well done mate, you passed the test!"

The filthy swine! Anyway, Al and the guitarist ended up doing a few lines of coke in the living room and I went into the kitchen and talked to his girlfriend. Eventually at about four in the morning, everyone collapsed on the sofas and I had my new best friend cuddled up next me, wagging his tail.

I got up at 7am and woke Al to tell him I was going and he told me to be careful just before I left the flat and walked back to my place. On the way there, I started to feel really weird and couldn't seem to judge distances properly. It wasn't drugs playing tricks with my head (I don't take them)

Making my way upstairs into the bathroom, I sat down on the toilet and couldn't breathe normally and started gasping for air, whilst holding on to the edge of the sink. The best way I can describe it was that the sensation was similar to being drunk but instead of having a muzzy head, my brain was going like a steam train and I was 100% focused (kind of like smoking a strong spliff but without the pleasant results)

I realise now that it was a panic attack but I'd had never had one before, so I was really scared. Still sitting on the toilet, I rang my brother Davey, who lived about eight miles away and told him that I wanted to go back into the hospital. I remember being absolutely terrified and he must have noticed it in the tone of my voice. He said he would come and pick me up because I was in no fit state to drive and would be about half an hour.

While I was waiting for him I started to feel so much calmer because I knew I was going back into hospital where they would look after me. It was more than that though; I now knew what John the DJ had meant when he said he liked it in there. I wouldn't say I liked it exactly; more that I felt safe and it was as if I was beginning to realise there may actually be something wrong with me. The panic attack had really shook me up and I had this overwhelming feeling that I was going to come to some harm. I don't mean that I was going to harm myself, it's like I could see my erratic behaviour was out of control and whereas I'd enjoyed it before, the sensation was now frightening me (big time!)

I missed Zee and Lucy and John, they knew how I was feeling and just being back in their company, I knew I would feel so much better. It's really weird but I actually couldn't wait to get back into hospital and this time I was prepared and packed a suitcase with my best suits, DVD's, CD's and portable speakers for my ipod. I was going to enjoy myself, especially as it was only four days away from Christmas!

When Davey and his partner Helen arrived, I remember letting them in and then giving them their Christmas presents as if everything was normal. I needed to take a quick shower and told them I wouldn't be long and when I was ready and it was time to go, I opened the front door and Darren the window cleaner was standing there.

"Hello John!" he said with a big smile on his face, "Where have you been?"

I couldn't help it and started to well up but didn't want him to see me like that so I turned my back on him and whispered to my brother, "Get rid of him, for fucks sake"

SECTION 2: MEDIUM

Walking back into my living room, I could hear Davey explaining to Darren, "I'm John's brother. He's coming to stay with us over Christmas and will be back soon. He's a bit busy at the moment," and then gently shut the front door, leaving Darren outside.
"Who's that?" asked Helen.
"He's a friend of mine," I replied. "He looks up to me a bit and I didn't want him to see me upset"
We could see Darren moving about outside and trying to look through the window but after about five minutes, he went away. Davey picked up my suitcase and put it into the boot of his car and I sat in the back seat. My landlord walked past and waved to me. I could tell by the look on his face that he knew something was wrong but I just smiled and waved back to him and then looked away.

CHAPTER 19

When we got to the hospital, I had to see two members of the crisis team, whose job it was to evaluate if a person should be in the hospital or not and to look out for their well being, once they were discharged. One of them was a black guy in his twenties and his name was Saviour and the other was a white lady in her thirties. I can't remember her name but there's no way it could ever compete with Saviour! They wanted to know why I felt I needed to come back into hospital after wanting to be discharged so quickly. I was upset and I could see my brother was too (he's quite a gentle person, bless and I love him to bits)

Davey described the panic attack I'd had and told them that he'd never heard me sound so scared on the telephone. They agreed I should be re-administered and after saying goodbye to my brother, Saviour led me back to my ward. I walked into the main hall, looking to see if Lucy was around but there was no sign of her and I guessed she must have been sleeping. I got my old bed back and after unpacking my stuff, went outside hoping to see Zee and John. Both of them weren't there and when I went back upstairs, I asked one of the nurses if they had seen them.

"Zee's gone shopping on his own as usual," he replied, "and John has been discharged"

"Oh right," I said and walked away. He'd been absolutely right, three days and then discharged!

SECTION 2: MEDIUM

A short while later I was getting myself a coffee, when I heard the main door open and close behind me.

"I don't fucking believe it! You must fucking really love it here!" roared Zee as he came over and patted me on the back.

I laughed and replied, "All right mate, been Christmas shopping?"

"Just stocking up on supplies, I'm going home to my mum's for a couple of days"

"That's great! Are you gonna get to see your son?"

"Yeah, his mum won't let him visit me here but said she'd bring him over to see me at my mum's house"

Zee had told me before that he'd met and married a concert pianist from Egypt and they'd had a son called Jake, who was now four years old.

God knows how he ever got to meet an Egyptian piano player, he never did tell me but he'd shown me a photo of her once and she was absolutely stunning. I looked down into the bag he was carrying and could see a big Teddy Bear.

"That for Jake?" I asked.

"Yeh, he'll fucking love it!"

"Does your wife still live in England then?"

"Nah, she fucked off back to Egypt when we split up. She's over for just a few days and then goes back for Christmas!"

"I bet you can't wait to see your boy"

"It's been over a year, I've almost forgotten what he looks like. Anyway, what you doing back here?"

"You know what it's like"

He put his hand on my shoulder. "Yeh, I know," he said.

"When you going?" I asked.

"Soon as my dad comes to pick me up. Where have they put you?"
"Back in the same bed"
"Make sure they keep my bed empty for when I get back," he said.
"How am I going to do that?"
"If they bring in anyone to our room, just tell 'em to fuck off!"
"Er yeh, okay. I'll see what I can do"

Zee left about an hour later and after going out into the courtyard for a cigarette, I got another coffee from the vending machine. When I turned around, I saw Lucy sitting down at one of the dining tables and she looked terrible and was just staring at the table top. She appeared to be completely spaced out and was as white as a sheet, so I walked over to the table and sat down opposite her.
"Hi Luce," I said.
She slowly lifted her head and looked into my eyes and through my eyes, through my head, into the wall behind me.
"I'm back"
She gave the faintest of smiles and then lowered her head again and I thought it best to leave her on her own so went to my room and lay down on my bed.
"Maybe it wasn't such a good idea coming back," I thought to myself. "John's been discharged, Zee's fucked off home for a few days and Lucy is on another planet!"
I must have dozed off for a couple of hours and when I woke up, I didn't have a clue where I was. Victor came into the room and told me that dinner was being served.

SECTION 2: MEDIUM

"Oh yeh, I know where I am" I told myself.

I got off the bed, walked over to the window and had a cigarette. Walking into the dining hall, I was surprised to see so many patients I didn't recognise because I'd only been gone two days. After queuing for my food, I sat down at an empty table and felt a tap on my shoulder.

"John, you're back!"

I recognised the voice immediately. "No, that's my shoulder," I replied.

Lucy looked totally different from before, almost back to her old self and I decided not to tell her that I'd already seen her earlier. She sat down next to me and actually put her hand on top of mine.

"I'm so pleased to see you John but why are you back?"

"I missed the food too much!"

Lucy started to laugh and then burst out crying. "I'm sorry," she sobbed, "I'm being selfish. I'm glad your back!"

I didn't reply, there was no need. I understood and she knew it.

"Shall we have our midnight chat tonight?" she asked while wiping her eyes with the back of her hand.

"Wouldn't miss it for the world!"

That night after the staff had given up trying to get us to bed, Lucy asked me if I was okay.

"My problems are nothing compared to yours," I answered.

She nodded slowly and remained silent, gently touching the scars on her left forearm.

"What's the matter Luce?"

"I've got to get out of here John; I can't stand it any longer"

"I know mate, well……… I think I know. It must be terrible for you. I can only imagine how you must be feeling"

"I've been here so long…….for ever! What have I done wrong?"

"You've done nothing wrong"

"It's when you were discharged the other day," she said and started to cry softly.

"What do you mean?" I asked and put my hand on her knee.

"Don't touch me!"

"I'm sorry"

She started to cry some more. "Don't be sorry John; it's not your fault. It's my fault!"

"No it isn't, it's that scumbag who raped you!"

Lucy stood up and wiped her eyes. "I'm going to bed John, goodnight"

"Night Lucy," I said as she walked away into the gloom, "don't do anything stupid"

She did not reply.

The next morning, I woke early and couldn't wait to get into the hall to see if Lucy was okay. To my relief, she was sitting at a table, eating breakfast with two other female patients. After grabbing some toast and a couple of sachets of jam, I sat down at a table with a few of the guys from my wing. I kept looking over at Lucy to see if she was alright but she kept her head down, as if concentrating on her food. When breakfast was over, we all queued for our meds and after spitting mine down the sink, I went over to the nurse's station and asked if I could go for a cigarette.

Lucy walked up slowly and she had that look where she was going to make a run for it. I put my back against the door release button to prevent her from pressing it and it was as if I wasn't even there. She walked right up to me, staring at the ground and with her head level with my chest. The staff in the nurse's station looked over in our direction and I gave them a reassuring nod.

"Don't do it Luce," I whispered, "It'll make things worse"

"How can things get any worse," she mumbled and looked up at me with tears in her eyes. I had to swallow hard to stop myself from crying, I will never forget the look on her face. I'm writing this over three years later and it's still choking me up thinking about it. A female orderly came out of the nurse's station.

"Are you ready John?" she asked.

"Ready," I replied and stood to one side, so she could press the button.

As she opened the door, Lucy started to follow us through.

"Not you Lucy, you know you haven't got any cigarettes left," said the orderly and I could see the muscles in Lucy's jaw, tighten.

"It's okay, she can have one of mine," I said.

"No, she's got to learn that once she's run out, she has to wait until she can afford to buy some more"

"She's a grown woman, stop fucking treating her like a little kid!"

"Mind your language John or you won't be permitted to have a cigarette"

While we were arguing, Lucy was slowly edging her way out the door and so the orderly stood in front of her, preventing her from going any further.

"This is a fucking joke!" I said, "If we were in the nick, there'd be a fucking riot if we weren't allowed to smoke!"

The orderly looked over to a male nurse, sitting at his desk and he gave a slight nod. Another female orderly came out of the nurse's station and told me to go on ahead as they both walked either side of Lucy. When we got outside into the courtyard, the two orderlies stood on the second step of the stairs leading up to the garden and I gave Lucy a cigarette and a light. She smoked it in silence and so I started speaking with the orderlies. They were both quite young and I thought, "What would they do if everything kicked off?"

As we were talking, Lucy dropped her cigarette and dashed towards the steps. Both orderlies immediately blocked her path and told her to go back down to where I was standing. I started to laugh, thinking it was just one of Lucy's feeble attempts at trying to escape but the orderlies obviously saw something I didn't. From experience, they could tell by Lucy's mannerisms that she was totally serious (I thought I knew her by now but they'd known her a lot longer than I had)

She tried to force her way through them and started screaming. Both the orderlies pinned her arms behind her back and even though she was small, they had to really struggle to keep her under control. They brought her down to her knees, so that her head was resting on the bottom step and Lucy screamed so loudly, it actually scared me. She wriggled like crazy and so they grabbed her hands and bent her wrists right back so the tops of her hands were touching between her shoulder blades, much the same as the police are taught to do.

"Come on Lucy, we're going back inside," one of them calmly stated.

SECTION 2: MEDIUM

Still with her wrists pinned up behind her back, they started to walk her towards the doors leading back into the building and for a second, she seemed to relax but then started thrashing about and screaming like a wild animal. My heart was pumping like mad; I was so worried for her but felt totally helpless.

"John, open the door!" one of them yelled out to me and as they walked inside, I followed them and shut the door behind me. As they were attempting to take her back up the stairs, Lucy managed to force her way over to the wall next to me, still with the orderlies holding onto her wrists. I felt like I had to do something and so I started to take hold of Lucy's upper arms when one of the orderlies shouted, "Get back John, we've got it under control!"

I was startled by the severity of her voice (she was only in her early twenties) and did exactly as I was told.

Lucy was bent forward and judging from the position her wrists were in, must have been in so much pain but that didn't stop her pulling herself right up to the wall and smashing her head against it, over and over again.

As I put my hand between her head and the wall, the other orderly pushed a panic button device they carried on their belts. Lucy's head slammed against my hand repeatedly and she was sobbing uncontrollably.

Mo, a male nurse who looked more like an overweight bank manager and wouldn't be capable of dealing with anything physical, came running down the stairs. He pushed the two orderlies out of the way and lifted Lucy up with one arm and told her that she was going back into Sherrin ward. He marched through the two doors opposite the ones leading to the garden, with

Lucy tucked under his arm and you could hear her screaming all the way down the corridor that led to Sherrin. The two orderlies and myself, stood at the bottom of the steps, out of breath and then I looked over to the youngest one and she said, "Now you know why I didn't want her going for a cigarette"

CHAPTER 20

I spent the rest of the day worrying about Lucy.
Tea time arrived and two male orderlies brought her into our hall and she was obviously drugged up to the eyeballs and was shuffling along with her head down. As she passed me, she looked up slightly and gave me a Malcolm McDowell smile and that made me feel so much better! That night, when everyone was asleep, I sat in my usual chair waiting for Lucy to come out for our evening talk but she didn't show.
The next morning and I was told that me and Maria had to have a blood test. Maria was the tall lady with the wild hair and the scary noises. Although I had been scared the first time I ever saw her, I could now see how vulnerable Maria was and my fears immediately vanished. A young nurse, who couldn't have been any more than eighteen, escorted us out of our ward, through the main entrance, across a car park, into the back door of the main hospital and down a service corridor which was full of pallets loaded with drugs and stuff. She pushed open this set of double doors and we found ourselves in another corridor, this time full of members of the public. As soon as Maria saw all these strange faces, she started to make her moaning noises again, so I held her hand and squeezed it gently, trying to reassure her that everything was okay. We followed the young nurse along the corridor and up a large spiral staircase which led to the main hospital reception and she looked on a large board and found the words "Blood Tests" with an arrow pointing

to the left. The three of us walked into the waiting room, which was packed with people and the nurse told us to sit down while she went to the reception desk. Maria was extremely anxious and squeezed my hand tightly, her groaning noises getting louder and louder. There were parents with their children waiting to see a doctor and they were all staring at us. I could see that the kids looked frightened (her noises were scary!) and were whispering to their parents who were trying to calm them down but you could see that they appeared to be concerned as well. We must have been sat there for fifteen minutes and I noticed our nurse waiting to be seen and not having any sense of urgency about her. I told Maria not to worry and that I would be back soon and went over to our nurse and told her to sit with Maria, which she did immediately (you have to appreciate that I was pumped up emotionally and was very intimidating)

I then walked past the reception desk, down this narrow corridor and straight into the doctor's room, where he was giving some woman a blood test. I told him that there were kids out there, terrified of the lady I was with and that we should be seen straight away! He replied that we had to wait our turn just like everybody else and carried on dealing with his patient.

"For fuck's sake!" I yelled and stormed out of his room, back to the waiting area where everyone was staring at me.

Our nurse looked totally confused and I told her to wait with Maria, while I went to these two security guards and explained what was going on. We went back to Maria and the nurse and I could see the doctor talking to the lady at the reception. She called over the security guards and our nurse and the doctor told her to take us back to our ward straight away. This is how badly run these places are! Don't get me wrong, everyone who works for the NHS in a caring or medical capacity deserves a medal but the management side of things is terrible! As soon as we got back to our ward, we were taken into the lady's wing and then into the meds room. One of our doctor's came in and gave us our blood tests. MENTAL!

Not only had they stressed Maria out big time but also scared loads of people in the hospital waiting room, when all they could have done is given us our blood tests in our own ward.

I had mixed feelings towards the staff from then on. One minute, I was angry with them for not doing things in a sensible way and the next minute, I had total respect for them because they were so caring. I came out of having my blood test and walked into the hall and Mo (the nurse who looked like a bank manager) was sitting at one of the dining tables, watching over the patients.

He liked to do crosswords at the same time and I went and sat with him. He was a really nice guy with a chilled out personality and a friendly way about him which was infectious.

"Been causing a spot of trouble have you John?" he said in a dry manner, without looking up from the crossword puzzle.

"This place is a joke," I replied, "why didn't they just give us our blood tests here?"

He put down his pen and looked up at me, "There wasn't a doctor available at the time," he said.

"They soon found one when I kicked up a fuss!"

"You have to appreciate John that this hospital, along with all the other NHS hospitals all over the country, are incredibly busy all year round"
"I understand that but so much time and upset could have been saved!"
He picked up his pen again and continued with the crossword. "You know what it's like," he said, "too many chiefs and not enough Indians"
I just shook my head and didn't reply.
Mo was a very religious man and we would have friendly disputes over god and all that malarkey and I would also help him do his crossword and he'd sulk when I knew an answer he didn't. His actual name was Morris Arleigh but everyone called him Mo after Mohammed Ali, even though he was white and I liked him a lot.

CHAPTER 21

Two days before Christmas, midday.

More and more patients were being admitted (busy time of year)
Zee was back and very agitated because apparently, he'd lost his temper whilst staying at his parents and so his wife refused to go round there with his son. We had a few games of pool and listened to the Floyd on the stereo. His favourite tune was "Welcome to the Machine" and in hindsight, I can see why. He'd spent all his adult life, in and out of institutions and had become like a coiled spring waiting to explode. I could tell that he wasn't his usual self because he was missing quite simple pots and he was a good player. He seemed to calm down after a while and asked Mo if he would walk him to the petrol station to buy some cigarettes. Since the argument with his parents, the staff had really come down heavy on him, saying that if he left the hospital unattended again, then he would be sent back to Sherrin ward.
While they were gone, lunch was being served and we all queued up to savour the al a carte cuisine! Everyone was sitting down eating their food, when Zee came storming back in and was clearly not very happy (to say the least!)
Mo followed behind and Zee started shouting at him about not being able to cross the road on his own.
"I ain't a fucking kid and don't need you to hold my hand!" he yelled.

Mo calmly tried to reason with him and Zee shouted out to everyone, "and his fucking name ain't MO, it's Morris..... MORRIS FUCKING ARLEIGH and he's a fucking prick!"

I tried not to laugh as Zee marched off into the games room and slammed the door behind him. The rest of us carried on eating our lunch, while Zee literally tore the games room apart. I could hear him swearing and breaking things up, so I got up, walked over to the games room door and looked through the glass. He had a pool cue in his hand and was using the butt of it to stab the surface of the table.

"Come back and sit down John!" called Mo and then he went into the nurse's station. He didn't even bother calling the Sherrin orderlies upstairs (they were all big burly brutes!) as he knew that even they would have had trouble controlling him! Ten minutes later, eight coppers stormed the games room and as I finished my desert, I thought to myself, "What's that terrible din?"

They dragged Zee out the games room with him swearing and screaming, out of the ward and down the corridor to the main exit. I followed them to their cars which were parked just outside, without anyone trying to stop me.

Zee was handcuffed and bundled into a back seat and as they drove off, he lifted his chained arms and waved to me. When I got back to our ward, I had the right hump because the games room door had a big padlock on it and through the window; I could see the pool table in ruins. That was my only bit of enjoyment, the dirty rat! Underneath all the debris, I could just see the stereo and more importantly, my "Wish You Were Here" album. Both seemed to have survived Tsunami Zee.

SECTION 2: MEDIUM

Lucy appeared to be improving and they even let her go outside for a cigarette. Whenever anyone wanted to smoke, one or two members of staff would always go with us. On this occasion, something really weird happened. They let Lucy go with me and this time, a member of staff didn't accompany us. While we were outside, I looked up at the window and saw Mo staring at us and he looked at me, nodded his head and then walked away. Everything any of the patients did was recorded in their files and they had obviously noted that me and Lucy spent a lot of time talking at night. Maybe they figured they'd have more luck with Lucy if there wasn't a member of staff accompanying her all of the time and could trust me to stop her from running away. I didn't really understand it but knew they weren't stupid and when Mo walked away from the window, he was obviously watching us from the CCTV cameras, hooked up to a monitor in the nurse's station. That afternoon I was due for an assessment by the psychiatrist and so wore one of my suits. My brother Davey attended and they asked the usual questions. We were on the first floor with two doctors and Victor, who was in charge of looking after me. The doctor asked if I still had strong protective feelings towards my sisters and I said that if anything happened to them, I would grab his car keys, jump through the window and drive down to see them. (Not the most sensible answer but hey, I was crazy!)
Needless to say, they did not discharge me.

After dinner that evening, my nephew Steve came to visit. He laughed when he saw me wearing a suit and I took him over to the padlocked games room door and told him to look through the glass. The pool table was in half, two cupboards were now nothing more than splinters of wood and the television on the counter, was now teetering precariously on the edge. I explained what had happened and Steve couldn't stop laughing. We went outside for a cigarette and I showed him how easy it was to just walk out of the place, by going up the steps to the garden and then opening the unlocked gate around the corner. As we were walking through the car park back to the front entrance of the hospital, he asked, "Why don't you run away?"

"And where am I gonna go," I answered, "I'm totally skint and wherever I go, they'll find me"

Steve's girlfriend was waiting by their car and after saying goodbye to them both; I went back inside and straight to bed.

Christmas Eve.

Everyone was still asleep. I got in the shower and started singing, "Oh What a Beautiful Morning" at the top of my voice. If I was awake, then so should everyone else be, ha ha!

I stepped out of the shower and two female nurses were in the corridor. This tiny little timid nurse looked at me in just a small towel and said that I shouldn't be walking around like that. I felt in high spirits and said to her, "This is the male wing, now get out! I feel violated!"

She scampered off and the other nurse smiled and shook her head and said, "You're a bad boy John"

Without Zee I was feeling lonely, him being next to me in our bedroom and all. There was this patient called John Barnet and he moved into Zee's bed. He was very intelligent but totally off his rocker and built synthesizers as a hobby and could play like Liberace on speed. He'd just come out of Sherrin and was convinced aliens were communicating to him through electric sound waves which were directly transported to his brain (told you)

The Polish doctor from my first night called me into his office and told me that I had to take my regular course of injections. I pointed out to him that he was looking at John Barnet's file, not John Barrett's. He looked at me sheepishly and said, "oh yes, er... this isn't your file"

"In your own time doc," I replied.

That evening Mo and a load of bible bashers doing the rounds, started belting out Christmas carols in the main hall. I was trying to watch the news and turned the T.V up full blast to drown out the awful singing.

Victor came over and turned it down.

I was dying for a fag and the festive racket wasn't helping any and I was starting to get seriously pissed off!

"We Wish you a Merry Christmas" started up and so I stood right next to the carol singers and started singing, "I wish I could have a fucking fag!" in the same tune. Mo finally gave in and told Victor to take me for a cigarette.

A guy called Chris had been there since I first came in and was I'm guessing, in his late forties. His daughter died of cancer, so he got drunk and crashed his car at 100mph and ended up with brain damage, the poor man. As a result, he became very abusive and would swear all of the time; it was almost like he was suffering from tourettes. During visiting time his wife told me that he used to be the friendliest and most polite person you could ever meet and as she spoke, I noticed that she looked totally exhausted. Not only had her daughter died but her husband ended up with brain damage. Chris started calling his wife a, "cheating bitch!" and Victor came over and quietly told him to calm down.

"FUCK OFF YOU BLACK CUNT!"

(That worked….not!)

He shouldn't have been in our ward or even sectioned because he wasn't mentally ill but brain damaged. His wife was battling with the hospital to get him transferred to a brain damage unit and to be fair to the staff, it wasn't their fault.

One of the female patients was a woman in her mid thirties who'd had some sort of breakdown. She was a very quiet lady and showed me photos of her three children who ranged from twelve years old, down to four. I remember when I had been initially discharged on my third day; she had cried and said that she hoped I would get better. She hardly even knew me but was such a kind and caring person and when I was readmitted, she seemed genuinely concerned for my well being. She said that her husband was picking her up in two hours time and she was going home for Christmas. "The doctor's said that if all goes well, then I won't have to come back"

Her husband had been looking after the children and although this was great news, I could tell she was worried about something.

"What's the matter?" I asked.

She started to cry and said she didn't want her children to see her like this because she felt ashamed and thought they might be scared of her. I felt so sorry for her, she was obviously a loving mother and wife and I gave her a big hug and said that they would understand. All of the time I had seen her on the ward, she was always wearing her dressing gown but now she was dressed smartly and I noticed a bag with presents in it, next to her chair. When her husband arrived to take her home, I was getting a coffee from the vending machine and when he put his arm around her, it really choked me up. During the rest of the time I spent on that ward, I never saw her again and only hope everything turned out okay for her. Because I couldn't play pool I went to my room, laid on the bed and listened to my ipod; 'Dark Side of the Moon' seemed to be the order of the day.

Christmas day.
Pissed off straight away. I'm not too keen on Christmas at the best of times and to be stuck in this place! My brother came to visit and had some presents and cards for me. He spent about half an hour with me and we talked about this and that. I could tell that he felt unfomfortable and that made me feel sad. At one point, I asked him if he could take me back to my flat so I could pick up some bits and pieces. He said that he couldn't because he was going over to Helen's dad's house for Christmas dinner and I got really pissed off with him. When he left, we were on quite bad terms and I feel so bad about it now. I thought that everything revolved around me and didn't consider the fact that other people had their lives to lead. Helen has a daughter and my brother is part of their family now. He'd found the time to come and visit me on Christmas morning and I wasn't even grateful. When he left, I needed a smoke and after I came back up, I

remembered the cards and presents Davey had brought with him. They were on one of the dining tables right outside the nurse's station and the young nurse, who took me and Maria to have our blood tests, said "Why don't you open them?"
I felt really angry inside and gave her a dirty look but when I saw the kind expression on her face, I nodded and said okay. The first card I opened was from my wife's sister and my brother-in-law. I ripped it in half. The next card was from my wife, same result. The next one was a handmade card from my daughter. I took it to my ward and put it next to my bed and cried and cried and cried myself to sleep (it was only 11am but I was already drained)

Timid little nurse prodding me.
I didn't know where I was for a moment.
She said that my wife and children were here to see me and so I got dressed straight away and went downstairs for a smoke to calm myself (by this stage, I could smoke whenever I wanted)
A female orderly called Tina took me out of our ward and through the main reception, into this room with paintings of animals and stuff all over it. My wife, youngest son and daughter were all sitting there. I asked where my eldest son was and my wife said that he didn't want to come. Those words were like a kick in the stomach but somehow, I managed not to break down. I sat opposite them and my daughter gave me a cup which she had painted (I still drink my tea out of it, to this day)
I told her that it was really lovely and asked her to look after it for me, as I didn't want it to get broken. I was really anti my wife (I don't know why) and asked

the orderly if she could wait outside. When she had gone, I couldn't think of anything to say to the kids and it felt so awkward. I asked them if they got any nice presents and that's all I could think of and so I said that maybe they should go now and I'll see them when I'm discharged. When they left I went back to my ward, pulled the curtain around my bed and cried myself to sleep.

Woke up at 5pm and walked into main hall.
Everyone was there and were all in good spirits. We had a great Christmas dinner and I felt a million times better! It made me appreciate how good the staff were because they all really made an effort to make it a nice occasion for the patients who hadn't gone home for the Christmas break. After dinner, Mo put on the radio over the intercom speakers and everyone seemed relaxed, even Chris was happy and refraining from swearing!!! Zoe's boyfriend (from my local pub) sent me a text, wishing me a Happy Christmas and hoped that I was okay. I replied that I was having a lovely time in this five star hotel and would see him when I got out. I sat next to Maria on one of the sofas by the TV and noticed that she wasn't making her scary noises. More to myself than anything, I started talking about what had happened to me over the past couple of months and Maria started to nod her head and say yes every so often. I held her hand and very quietly she said that she had owned a boutique in Marbella, selling very expensive dresses and drove a top of the range BMW. Her business had been going from strength to strength and she got introduced to this guy at a party one night. They started to see each other and he got her into coke in a big way. As she told me this,

I suddenly realised why she kept putting her hand to her nose, over and over again. I just thought it was a nervous thing but now it all made sense. Her parents and sister who were very wealthy lived quite near to the hospital and were extremely worried about her. As she spoke to me, I looked at her properly for the first time and realised just how attractive she was and I could imagine when she was okay, how glamorous she would have been. Meds time and Maria was up like a shot (she loved her medication!)

Mo had been sitting at a table nearby while me and Maria were talking. He strolled up to me and sat down.

"That's the first time I've ever heard her speak" he said.

CHAPTER 22

Funny, what started off as such a rotten day ended up being one of the best Christmas days I've ever had............ and there wasn't even any booze to hand! The ward phone rang later that evening and I picked it up (staff were not allowed to answer, just us loonies)
"Hello, Ping Pong's Chinese take-a-way, can I take your order?" I said.
"John! It's Jane"
Jane is my youngest sister (two years older than me) I'm the baby of the family and she lives in Sydney. It was great to speak to her and I think she was surprised at how cheerful I was sounding. I remember asking her to contact my eldest son, to see if she could get him to visit or at least ring me and she promised she would.

One o'clock in the morning and me and Lucy were up as usual, when Victor brought in a new guy called Luke. He reminded me of a young Robert Redford who hadn't washed for about a week and had long hair and a stubble (a bit hard to imagine, I grant you)
Victor told me and Lucy to go to bed as usual and we ignored him as usual. Luke paced up and down the room, telling everyone and no one (me and Lucy were the only ones up) about the fucked up government and how Jesus would solve everything! Lucy looked at me and rolled her eyes as if to say, "Here comes another one!"

You have to imagine that after 11pm, all the lights were turned off except for the ones in the nurse's station, so it could be quite eerie in the hall with a new bloke wandering about, spreading the word of the lord (Halleluiah)

Eventually, Victor came out and steered Luke off to bed. Lucy was in a talkative mood and I could sense there was something she wanted to tell me. I didn't push it but listened to all her stories of self-harm and years of being sectioned. Of course it was terrible to be raped by that cab driver but I sensed that she was a strong person deep down and so asked her if there was something else that had happened to her? She held my arm (which was VERY unusual) as she didn't like any physical contact. I have a habit of patting people on the shoulder to comfort them and whenever I did it to Lucy, she would say, "DON'T TOUCH ME!"

There was only one man that she would allow to touch her and that was her fiancé Stewart. Turns out that Stewart went around all the nut houses and comforted the distressed with readings from the scripture (praise the lord!)

You can probably tell by now that I'm not a religious person but on meeting Stewart, I had the utmost respect for him because he was a thoroughly decent man. If it were not for him, Lucy would still have been in Sherrin!

Needless to say, Lucy was religious too and if that's what it took to give her strength then fair play. She whispered to me that about a year before the cab driver incident, her dad had gone into her bedroom in the middle of the night when her mum was asleep and started to hug her, then kiss her and then he raped her.

SECTION 2: MEDIUM

Lucy could see that I was boiling inside and whispered to me, "Don't worry John, it's no big deal"
No big deal! That bastard had ruined her life and still lived happily at home with his loving wife, while Lucy's life was in ruins! She sat there quietly, all peaceful like and waited for me to calm down and actually asked me if I was alright? (Love you Lucy, you're my hero!)
Suddenly I felt really tired and asked if she minded if I went to bed. I think that seeing my kids and listening to so many sad stories, had taken its toll on me.
"Of course not" she replied.
I got up and kissed her on the top of her head and as I walked back to my bed I realised that she had let me touch her. I felt so privileged and slept like a log!

Boxing Day.
Had a lie in and got up late (7am)
I walked into the main hall and grabbed a coffee or ten from the vending machine. Luke appeared and seemed to be confused.
"All right mate?" I called out.
He rattled on about god while I chatted up the nurse (in my best whistle)
John Barnet wandered out and he and Luke had some weird conversation about aliens landing on earth 2000 years ago and one of them was Jesus or something. Who cares, I was in with the nurse! You have to remember that I was on a massive high at this stage, the BIG low followed but you might want to skip that bit, it's fucking depressing! Mo took me, John Barnet and Luke downstairs for a cigarette. John and Luke didn't have any fags; they just wanted to share the end of mine and then any stubs in the ashtray.

BIPOLAR.....ME?

I remember being shocked by this at the time but now know people who do it on a daily basis! (but more about that in another book)

Back upstairs and Ennio was awake and wandering around. He couldn't speak a word of English and was only 19. His parents paid for him to come over from Italy to try as a striker for some big football team (I can't remember which one, I'm not a big football fan)

He had a trial for this team and was at Stanstead Airport, waiting to go home when he had a major breakdown. No one trying to help him could speak Italian and so they called the police and he ended up here! The management were trying to organise his flight home and into an Italian hospital, via the Italian embassy but it was taking ages (red tape!)

In the men's wing, there were three single bedrooms for people whom the doctor's felt it would be beneficial to have their privacy.

1st bedroom: Ennio, who would scream all night long. (I felt so sorry for him, in a madhouse in a foreign country and couldn't express his feelings to anyone)

2nd bedroom: Craig, a public schoolboy who went on a school trip to Austria and the teachers let the kids do want they wanted while they all got pissed. He took an ecstasy tablet and had a bad reaction and then tried killing himself. It was his friends who had to take him to the hospital because all the teachers were wasted! I asked him if the teachers got the sack and he said that the school covered it all up. I was so angry! This poor boy ended up in this place while those fuckers kept their jobs!

3rd bedroom: Nigel, a bank manager for Barclays (about sixty) and a terrific bloke. The recession kicked in and he was snowed under with loan requests.

SECTION 2: MEDIUM

Because he was such a decent man, the loan applicant's woes got to him and he had a breakdown. His wife took him to a hospital and while they were waiting to see a doctor, she went to the toilet and he threw himself off the roof and broke both his legs (I suppose he was lucky in a way, medical attention not being too far away!)

A few days earlier I had lent Ennio my iPod as I thought this would be a good way of me getting to communicate with him, music being universal and all that jazz (or rock or pop or soul)
He loved the music I had and I let him keep hold of the iPod until either of us was discharged first. Because of my bipolar, I felt I was indestructible; everything I did was the right thing to do and I knew better than anybody else. This woman walked in to the main hall and said that she ran a music group and would anyone like to join in.
"Yeh, why not," I thought to myself, "There's nothing else to do"
That afternoon, she walked in with all these percussion instruments and loads of patients from other wards. We all went into our games room and sat in a circle and were given the choice of a certain drum to play. I picked what looked like the loudest thing and found two paint sticks on the worktop. (I've never played drums in my life and started to play)
This woman started laughing and encouraged everyone to join in. I never realised I had a musical ear until then and was really surprised how well I was doing. A guy opposite started to grin and then played like lightening on his own drum. He had one of those military type drums and I asked him to do a

drum roll. Wow, that man was fast! I got chatty with him and he told me that he was an extra on TV, Eastenders being his most regular work. Look out for a big man on a stall in the market, that's the fella. I don't watch it myself but I'm sure he was telling the truth. After the class, he said that he teached music as his main job and that he'd teach me how to play guitar (my favourite) for free! He gave me his card and I lost it............. SHIT! I never saw him again as he was in another ward on another floor.

At last, a translator was brought in for Ennio, so he could finally talk to the doctors. I was so pleased for him but Luke and John were starting to piss me off. They followed me everywhere and copied everything I did (even down to shaving all their hair off!)
Luke kept sprouting on about the "fucking government man, they cover everything up man" and all that usual bollocks! I was really missing Zee but there was a rumour going round that he was in Sherrin and could be coming up to our ward soon. After dinner and meds (I was still spitting them out or giving them to Luke to make him docile and hopefully shut him the fuck up!) I sat next to Maria who seemed all chilled out. I'd asked Ennio (via the translator) if I could have my iPod for a few hours and he reluctantly agreed. I scrolled down the menu and found "Fun City" by John Barry, put one earplug headphone thingy in Maria's ear and the other in mine. As John B. tickled the ivories, Maria shut her eyes and whispered to herself, "Hmmm, that's nice"
I knew she would like it, she was a classy dame!
The other guy in my bedroom (who slept a lot) was called Derek. He had greased back hair (D.A. style)

and wore a teddy boy suit. Derek was in his mid to late forties and had thick lensed glasses. Obviously an early Elvis fan and all things rock and roll but his absolute favourite song was, 'What Do You Want to Make Those Eyes at Me For?' by Emile Ford. On my first full day in the hospital, in between waiting to see a doctor or nurse, I walked into the quiet room and noticed some CD's next to a player. I looked through them and noticed they were all rock and roll songs and so put one in and pressed play. Through the glass window, I could see Derek staring at me and his arm began to shake (as it always did when he was agitated) I could tell that by playing his music, it annoyed him (they were obviously his own C.D's) and so I turned the volume up for a laugh. His face was now beginning to go red with rage and for some reason; I suddenly got the feeling that he was a decent man. I stopped the player and took the C.D out and carefully put it back in its case. I then went out of the quiet room and sat in an armchair in the main hall. Derek walked towards the quiet room (still giving me the evil eye) and picked up all of his C.D's and went back to his bed. Over the next few days, me and Derek became friends (when he was awake that is) and I only hope he is ok now. His liver was completely ruined through drink and he refused to have a transplant. Melanie my advocate was very close to Derek and she told me that he could die at any moment. I mention Derek at this point because while I was listening to the iPod with Maria, I could see Ann watching Songs of Praise on the T.V. Now Ann really pissed me off because she was a stuck up bitch who clearly didn't like me (I could just tell)

She was in her sixties and looked down her nose at everyone. The only person she seemed to get on with was Nigel (the hospital roof jumper!) and that's only because he was such a gentleman, he wouldn't tell her to go and shove it! Derek slept all day and usually got up at about eight in the evening. He missed Christmas day completely and nurses had to wake him up to give him his meds and then he went straight back to sleep again. I saw Derek walk into the hall wearing his dressing gown and listening to his walkman. He was singing his favourite song and I noticed Ann glaring at him.
"Shut up!" she yelled.
"Altogether now!" I shouted, "So what do ya wanna make those eyes at me for, if they don't mean what they say!"
Derek grinned like a Cheshire cat and I got up and stood next to him so I could hear the music through his headphones. In unison, we sang at the top of our voices while staring straight at Ann. She got up and stormed off into the lady's wing and I thought to myself, "Go on, fuck off you stuck up bitch!"
Out of the corner of my eye, I noticed Victor in the nurse's station trying not to laugh.

1am, 27th December.

Me and Lucy were talking in the darkness.
BANG!
The door burst open and in marched Amy Winehouse.
"What the fuck?!"

CHAPTER 23

"I fucking hate you, you cunt, you fucking selfish bitch. You're a fucking cunt!"
This girl who was the absolute spitting image of Amy Winehouse came storming into the hall and Victor turned a couple of lights on. She was followed by her mum and dad and it was mum who was getting all the verbal abuse. Me and Lucy were convinced it was the real Amy, she was so alike and this was the place where you would expect her to end up. Victor was about 18" inches taller than this girl and he calmly went over to her and put a reassuring hand on her shoulder.
"Get the fuck off me nigger!" she screamed and Victor smiled and gently took his hand away.
"This is gonna be interesting," I whispered to Lucy and she just nodded her head.
No one had actually noticed we were there as the lights were off in our little corner. Amy 2's mother looked at Victor and said, "I am so sorry"
Victor smiled that great smile of his and said, "It's ok."
"Don't fucking apologise to that nigger you bitch!"
I noticed that her dad stood back a little and didn't say a word; I think he was in shock. It turned out her name was Dominique and she was 21.
Victor looked towards her mum and dad and said that it would be best if they left. Dominique's dad gave her a kiss on the cheek and when her mum tried to do the same, she pushed her away and told her to fuck off.

They slowly walked out of the hall with Dominique's dad comforting the mum who was in a right old state. Victor stood there staring at Dominique and when she told him to, "Fuck off you nigger cunt!" he smiled and slowly walked back to the nurse's station and sat down, watching her through the glass while doing some paperwork.

She got herself a coffee, slumped down in a chair and started singing and it was at this point I realised that she was definitely not the real Amy Winehouse. Me and Lucy sat quietly and just watched her and she was completely unaware we were even there. Luke came out of his bedroom and got himself a coffee. He sat down at the table with Dominique and asked her if she was okay. She said yes and carried on singing without even looking at him. Luke stared at her and she suddenly got up and shouted, "and NO, I'm not Amy FUCKING Winehouse!" and then started to wander around the hall.

Luke said nothing; he just stared into his coffee. Dominique started to walk in our direction and Lucy whispered, "Fag time I think"

"Not yet," I replied.

Dominique spotted us in the gloom and came over and stood in front of us. We both didn't know what to say and so we just stared at her.

"What are you looking at?" she said.

I thought for a moment and replied, "Not Amy Fucking Winehouse, that's for sure"

With that, she burst out laughing and sat down next to us. The light above us went on and in the nurse's station; Victor seemed pretty chilled (come to think of it, he was always pretty chilled!)

SECTION 2: MEDIUM

She started to sing the same song again and looked at me.
Singing. "What's your name?" Singing.
"John"
Singing. "I'm Dominique" Singing.
She turned to Lucy, singing, "What's your name?" Singing.
Lucy got up and walked off back to her room.
"What the fuck is wrong with that crazy bitch?"
I got up and went to bed, leaving Victor doing his paperwork, Luke staring into his coffee and Dominique singing, singing, fucking singing!

I woke up at 6am and walked into the main hall. Luke was asleep on one of the sofas so I went into the laundry room to get a blanket and covered him up. Dominique was nowhere to be seen, she probably stayed up half the night ranting and raving. I said good morning to Victor whose shift ended in an hour. He gave me a cigarette and a lighter and I went downstairs for a smoke or three (I had two stashed)
When I walked back upstairs to our ward, I saw a boy of seventeen with his mum and dad. He seemed to be drugged up and was sitting with Victor and Nelson who was just about to start his shift. Nelson was also African and he usually worked with Davina, a white nurse in her thirties. Davina would sometimes work extra shifts and when Nelson left at four, Tina would start. Tina was an orderly and features quite a lot in the LOW section of the book and you'll be hearing a lot about her soon. Chris (the brain damaged man) entered the hall and started ranting about his 'fucking slut of a wife having an affair with his best friend' (none of it was true)

I overheard the boy's dad asking if there was a child ward for his son and Nelson said that unfortunately they didn't have a child section but they would look into having him transferred to a different hospital as soon as possible. Over the past few days, word had spread around that I was a decent player on the pool table. Melanie my advocate had kindly donated the one Zee obliterated (she was not happy about that, I tell you) but luckily, Sherrin had a spare one. They got through a lot of tables in Sherrin! After lunch the previous day, I'd been playing pool with Ennio when two of the biggest black orderlies I had ever seen, walked into the room (they looked like a couple of fucking bouncers!) and had come up from Sherrin (where else)

"Which one's John?" one of them growled.

"Me"

They both looked at Ennio and he got the message and left the room mid game. I set up the balls again and slaughtered the first brute. It was touch and go with the second orderly but they both left eventually with their tails between their monstrous legs! So now, I walked up to Maz (17 year old kid) and patted him on the shoulder and introduced myself. I asked him if he would like a game of pool and he looked up at me with sad but friendly eyes and said that he didn't know how to play.

"Go on Maz" said his dad and so he got up and we walked into the games room, giving his mum and dad the opportunity to speak to Victor and Nelson in private.

I set up the balls and explained a few things to Maz regarding the rules and told him that I would break, that way I could then show him which would be the best ball to pot. As I watched him timidly take his shot, I realised that I had a son a year older than him, whom with my other son and daughter, I missed so much. Maz missed the ball he was trying to pot and he looked at me and said sorry. I warmed to him immediately.

"You don't have to apologise," I said and over the next half an hour, I noticed him improve greatly and his confidence increase. Eventually his mum and dad came into the games room and watched us play for a while.

I asked Maz's dad if he would like to play his son and Maz immediately said no and that I should play him instead. As we were playing, I talked to both Maz's parents and they were such nice people who looked physically and mentally drained. I felt that I would win the game and so decided to miss a few pots but knew that if he was 100% back on track; Maz's dad would have beaten me. It came down to the black and I missed the pot. Quietly, Maz said, "come on dad" and sure enough, he potted the winning ball. His mum stood up and I could tell it was time for them to go and so I told Maz that I'd see him in a minute and left the quiet room, saying goodbye to his parents.

"Oh shit! I'd forgotten about her"

Dominique appeared from the lady's wing, all bleary eyed and in a foul mood. The hall was busying up and she turned around to everyone and no one and yelled, "You fucking weirdo's, I don't belong here! HELLO, can anybody hear me?"

Nobody answered and I decided to keep my distance so went to get some breakfast and walked past Luke who was sitting up with the blanket wrapped around him, rubbing his newly shaved head. I sat there eating my brekkies and watched Dominique push her face against the nurse's station window yelling, "Can you hear me, you fucking pricks, let me out!"

I just laughed and thought to myself, "You're going nowhere, you mad bitch!"

At that moment, Zee walked through the main door. His voice was as deep as I'd remembered as he called out, "I'm back, have you all missed me?"

Dominique turned away from the window and walked straight up to Zee.

"I'm Dominique, who are you?"

"I don't give a fuck who you are, now what's for breakfast? I'm fucking starving!"

It was good to have him back!

Dominique muttered something like, "prick!" under her breath and went and slumped herself down on one of the sofas.

"YOU FUCKING LOUD MOUTHED CUNT!" screamed Chris and then went quietly back to his frosties.

Dominique said nothing and I looked over to Lucy who was sitting alone and saw her smile.

"MEDICATION TIME"

We all queued up as usual except for Dominique of course.

"I'm not taking any of that fucking shit!" (Such a charming girl)

Nelson and Davina walked over to her and gave her the same routine, "If you won't take your medication orally, we will have to administer it by injection"

"Lethal hopefully" I thought to myself.

"Fuck you, you're all a load of cunts. You're not coming anywhere near me with a fucking needle!"

SECTION 2: MEDIUM

"Stupid bitch! She'll learn" whispered Zee in front of me in the queue.
"I doubt it somehow," I replied.
Sure enough, five minutes later, two Sherrin orderlies came in, accompanied by a doctor I had never seen before.
"Ok mate?" one of the orderly's called out to Zee.
"Not bad son, not bad"
They walked towards Dominique.
"Keep the fuck away from me, you cunts!"
One orderly grabbed her legs and the other under her arms and they carried her off to the lady's wing, followed by the doctor brandishing the needle.
"CUNTS, FUCKING FUCK FUCK, CUNTING FUCK CUNTS!"
(You get the general idea)

After meds (John Barnet had mine) me and Zee went for a fag, unaccompanied. Because Zee had been in the system so long, they knew he was at a mellow stage and dependant on the hospital and so would not try to break out. He'd been in institutions since a teenager and had been in Cranbridge Hospital, before they knocked it down and turned the site into one of these poncy private gate entranced places, full of these houses trying to look like they were built 100 years ago. (Who gives a fuck about the patients; we've got a load of footballers with money to burn, who need somewhere to show off to some blonde bimbo!)
He had been in there the same time as my advocate Melanie and the stories they told me, made this place look like Butlins. Cranbridge was one of those old Victorian institutions and by the things I heard, had not changed much from Vicky's time on the throne!

He told me that the first time he had come to this hospital, they had put him in our ward and after a few months, discharged him. He went back to his mum's and begged her to get in contact with his wife, who was living back in Egypt with their baby son. When she tried but failed to make contact, he started to lose the plot and so called a cab to take him back to hospital. When the cab pulled outside the entrance, Zee got out and told the driver he didn't have any money. The cabbie wasn't too pleased with this and threatened to call the police. Zee started swearing at him and pushing him through the open window and so the cab driver grabbed a baseball bat from under his seat and hit Zee across the arm. Zee grabbed the man by the throat and in his own words, "I tried to rip out his jugular!"

Luckily for the cabbie, five orderlies came rushing out and dragged Zee off of him and took him down for a six month stay at Hotel Sherrin.

Zee is one of those people who can't hide their emotions and when angry, lets them out for all to see (and feel!)

When we went back upstairs, I noticed that Lucy was not around (strange that she hadn't come for a cigarette) and must have gone back to her room. I got this feeling that although it had been only a few hours since they met, she couldn't stand to be in the same room as Dominique.

I introduced Maz to Zee.

"Alright son, how ya doing?"

The three of us spent the next hour playing pool and I soon realised that Maz was a real hustler and could play after all; in fact he was so good that he beat Zee who jokingly threatened to smash his face in with a

SECTION 2: MEDIUM

pool cue. We all had a laugh and told Maz to have a go in the massage chair. That thing was fucking brilliant! Think of a dentist chair but instead of just going up and back, it vibrates and pummels you all over the bleedin' place!

Maz was in his glory and we said that if he wanted to lie on his front, we would leave the room!

Since the destruction of the games room, the door always had to be jammed open whenever Zee was in there. About an hour until lunch and as Zee took his shot on the black; I heard the release button sound to the main door.

I looked down, Zee potted the black.

I looked up and saw through the door, a woman walking into the hall.

I looked at Zee and he was all smug.

I looked at the woman.

I'd seen her somewhere else before......

Myra Hindley! Shit!.............could it get any worse?

CHAPTER 24

Davina and Ann (the stuck up bitch) were setting the tables and I saw Nelson helping Myra Hindley to sit down at one of the dining tables. I found out eventually that her name was Sarah, although I don't remember speaking to her or her speaking to anyone else. She didn't look like Myra Hindley from that infamous photo with bleached hair but when she was in prison, later on with brown hair.

Because he beat me on the last game, I asked Zee if he wanted to play the best of three. I won the second and so we were now on the deciding game. Davina stuck her head through the open doorway and said that it was time to sit down for our lunch.

"Five minutes luv," bellowed Zee.

He went on to beat me and so I said that we'd have to play again later on.

Me, Maz and Zee got some food and sat at a table behind Chris, Ann and Sarah (Myra)

Owing to where I was sitting, I was facing Sarah's back and she seemed to be in some sort of a trance. While Zee was talking to me, I watched as Sarah picked up her knife and holding it under the table, she clenched her fist around it as tightly as possible. I made a mental note to tell Nelson and to keep my distance!

Dominique refused to, "EAT THIS FUCKING SHIT!" and rang her dad up on her mobile.

SECTION 2: MEDIUM

"I DON'T CARE IF YOU'VE ALREADY LEFT, GO BACK AND GET ME SOMETHING FUCKING DECENT TO EAT!"

Zee looked over to her and said, "Shut the fuck up, I'm trying to eat over here!"

Nelson told Zee to calm down and he muttered something under his breath. After lunch, the usual mob went for a smoke. Because we had Luke and John Barnet with us, two orderlies came along too. I got to meet other patients from a different ward when we went outside and on this occasion, there was a girl who was probably in her early twenties. She was a nervous wreck and kept mumbling something about her husband. Melanie my advocate came down for a crafty fag and stood in the blind spot, so the staff upstairs couldn't see her on the CCTV. She was a brilliant person and I had so much respect for her. Luke and John were doing the usual rummaging through the ashtray thingy and were begging me for a cigarette. I was running a bit low myself and so gave them only one to share. Thankfully, Dominique didn't smoke. Five minutes peace!

Melanie comforted this nervous girl and when her orderly took her back to her own ward, she told me that on the day before she was going to be married, the groom told her that he was seeing someone else and wanted to call off the wedding.

When we went back upstairs, Dominique was in the games room with Maz and Craig (the public schoolboy) who was playing on his Xbox. You were allowed to bring your own electrical equipment in to the hospital but it had to be P.A.T tested before you could use them. I was still waiting for my laptop speakers (powerful!) to be done and in the meantime, I plugged my iPod into Derek's stereo. Maz asked me if I wanted a game and I decided to teach the young whipper snapper a thing or two. I eight balled the poor lad and then told him to play Zee. Dominique was in the massage chair (getting her rocks off) and singing that bleedin' song again and Lucy walked in and sat in a chair in the corner. Zee beat Maz and then set them up for me to play.

As I was about to break (with my back to the open door) Sarah shuffled in with her head down in total silence. It's like she was sleepwalking or had been hypnotised or something. I stood up straight and waited for her to go past me. She walked slowly around the pool table, shuffling her feet and stood next to Lucy and looked out of the window with her back to everyone. We all stared at each other and even Dominique didn't say anything (she even stopped singing that bloody song!)

Resting my chin on the pool cue, I broke and was fully aware whenever my back was against Sarah until she eventually turned around and shuffled back outside. Lucy looked at me with a pained expression on her face (it was like some kind of telethapy) she could feel and understand this other woman's suffering.

"Oi mate, what you in here for?" called Dominique to Craig.

He didn't reply and didn't turn around.

"Fuck you then," she muttered quietly, under her breath.

Calmly, Zee told her to leave him alone and asked why she was here. She got out of the massage chair and leant against the pool table, scattering the balls in the process.

SECTION 2: MEDIUM

"Fucking great!" I thought to myself, "I was winning as well"

"What is it with you fucking lot?" she asked, "No one fucking answers me!"

"Everyone in here has got their own problems and want to keep them private," replied Zee.

She told us all that she'd supposed to be have been going on a cruise with a load of mates to the Caribbean today but her parents had stopped her and brought her here. I told her that she should at least pretend to take her meds and dispose of them ASAP but she didn't listen, she just kept rattling on about herself. It turned out that she went to the same drama school as the real Amy Winehouse but was in the year below. The song she kept singing was her own composition and I didn't have the heart to tell her that it was absolute crap! Her and a few friends started doing pole dancing to earn some extra money and she decided to set up her own company, hiring out girls to dance at different clubs. She convinced her dad to convert an outbuilding where they lived in an expensive part of Essex, into a dance studio, with three poles, music system, mirrors etc. I started to get bored and told Zee that I was going for a fag. Usually Zee would have joined me but this time, he stayed (I think he fancied her)

Lucy stood up and said she would come but I pointed out that it was not her allotted time to smoke. She slumped back in the chair, crossed her arms and sulked.

Dinner Time.

Me, Maz, Zee and Dominique sat together. Lucy sat with Sarah and Maria. Dominique refused to eat; she was waiting for her dad to bring, "SOME PROPER FUCKING FOOD!"

Visiting time was in one hour and by this time, Nelson had finished his shift and Tina had taken over. Tina had such a kind and pretty face and was so caring towards all of the patients. She was everyone's favourite member of staff and I found myself starting to fancy her.

Before I was sectioned the first time around, I had bought loads of Christmas presents for all the people I knew. It didn't matter if I had only just met them; they were on my Christmas list!

When my brother collected me to go back into hospital, I took all the presents with me. I knew that I was going to be in there over the Christmas period and so would give the presents to the guys on my ward.

There was this brilliant gift shop where I lived and that's where I did most of my Christmas shopping. I bought these three brightly coloured clay models of African safari animals and I began to think that each one represented someone on my ward. I gave Craig a giraffe because he seemed so elegant and harmless, Dominic (whom I'll mention soon) a rhino because he was stocky and self assured and Tina a lioness because I thought I was falling in love with her. As a result of my bipolar disorder, money was no object and so I would spend a lot on gifts. My favourite perfume is Joy and I bought the biggest bottle available. For my two sons I got Sony digital photo frames and for my daughter, I purchased an iPod and speakers. Before being admitted into hospital, I had bought two front row tickets for The Nutcracker Suite showing at The Royal Opera House in Covent Garden. They were a Christmas present for Bee and myself to go and see

and were dated for early January. I had given them to Bee the last time I saw her and told her to look after them. I'd started getting into ballet (not too seriously) after seeing the film 'The Red Shoes'
I absolutely love that film and am a big fan of Powell and Pressburger movies.
One Saturday before I had been sectioned, I needed to get a new battery for my best watch and so drove to the next village to get it fitted. When I was walking back to my car, I noticed an amateur art exhibition was showing in the village hall, for local artists. I spent about an hour looking at all of the paintings and as I was leaving, the lady at the desk asked me if I would take part in writing down my favourite picture as the eventual winner would get a cash prize. I said I would and went back to a painting of a ballerina which I thought was great. I took a good long look at it and decided that it should be my choice as best picture. To be fair to the other artists though, I thought they were all great but I had to choose one.
Driving back to my flat, I couldn't get that image of the ballerina out of my mind and decided that I had to have it and so drew some money out, returned to the village hall and bought it. When I got back home, I put it up in the downstairs loo and stared at it for ages. The name and telephone number of the artist was on the back of the painting and a few days later, I gave her a call and eventually purchased a further two ballerina paintings off this lady and I love them to bits. I also bought two C.D's of The Nutcracker Suite, one for me and the other for Bee so we could become familiar with the music.

CHAPTER 25

For a forty two year old man I was relatively naive when it came to relationships with women (I'd been with my wife since the age of 19) and because of my bipolar disorder I felt as if any woman being at least the tiniest bit friendly towards me, wanted to start up a relationship. Ever since Ennio had started screaming in the night, he had been placed on suicide watch and that meant a member of staff would have to take it in turn to sit outside his room, not only at night but whenever he was in his bedroom (which was about 80% of the time)

Whenever Tina was on watch I would flirt with her and mess about by pulling silly faces through the windows in the connecting doors to my wing.

I mentioned Dominic (the rhino)

Well come to think of it; he had his own bedroom too, so there must have been four private rooms, not three. I'm guessing he must have been in his early thirties and had a well paid job working on the print. He was a really cool dude who had this great way about him, quiet but not at all shy (he just kept himself to himself) but you knew that he could handle himself. Coke was his downfall too but that didn't stop him taking it still whenever he was allowed out for a couple of hours, every other night.

(Something I wasn't allowed to do)

Before I had been admitted, he'd become involved with a girl from the women's wing and since she had been discharged, he would go round to her place at

every opportunity, when he was allowed out. They would do a couple of lines and then.... (well, you can guess what they did next)
It's funny but even though I've changed the names of most of the people in this book to respect their privacy, I still don't like to disclose more than I have to. After I was eventually discharged myself, I saw them both at the local shopping centre and it made me realise that you can walk past people every second of every day and not know the trauma's some of them have had to endure. All I will say is that Dominic was a top, top man and I hope his life is back on track.

After dinner, I went for a smoke with Luke and John buzzing around me like flies as per usual. I came back up and saw that Dominique had visitors, her mum and dad and two of her friends. She had obviously been phoning them non-stop because they had brought a lot of stuff with them. She finally got to eat (some pasta thingy and trendy yoghurt for desert)
Chris's wife walked in (looking completely knackered) and was met with the usual torrent of abuse! Craig's mum and dad were there also and they were allowed to go into his bedroom. I said hello to Maz's parents and they went and sat down in the corner by the T.V.
I sat on my own watching all the visitors and someone called my name.
My cousin Mick and his wife Pauline were standing there and I was so surprised to see them. I mentioned my cousin Lee, who left work that time to come and see me; well Mick is his dad and he is actually my cousin (It's just that Lee is nearer to my age and it get's very complicated going into second cousins and all that stuff)

They both sat down with me and it was so great to see them. I can't actually remember what we talked about but why we were in the middle of a conversation, Dominique got up from her table (leaving her family and friends) and came and sat with us and started introducing herself to Pauline and Mick. They looked at me a bit awkwardly and I asked Dominique politely, if she wouldn't mind letting us have some time in private. She didn't get nasty but I could tell that she didn't like it. Luckily, her friend came over and asked her to come back to their table. This seemed to do the trick and as Dominique left, her friend said sorry to us and then I looked over to her dad and he gave an apologetic nod to me. Finally, Mick and Pauline had to go and me and my big cousin hugged each other (a very rare thing for two Barrett men to do! Ha ha) and Pauline gave me a kiss. When they were gone, Maz called me over and I sat down with him and his parents. I told them how Maz had tricked me into thinking he was a novice pool player and his dad laughed, saying that he had been in the army and become very adept at the game and taught Maz everything he knew! While we were talking, I noticed Zee on his own and said to Maz that he should offer him a game. Zee accepted and they both went off to the games room. While he was gone, Maz's mum and dad told me that he had attempted suicide on numerous occasions and both of them felt so guilty because they somehow felt it was their fault. I may be wrong but I sensed that Maz's dad felt partly to blame because he'd spent so much time away from home, his son had somehow thought he didn't care about him.

SECTION 2: MEDIUM

Visiting time over, just us loonies left alone.
The doctors had so much faith in Lucy's fiancé Stewart; they'd allowed her to go home with him for the night. Very selfish of me but although it was great for Lucy, it meant I didn't have my talking partner for the evening.
Dominique was noticeably subdued that night, I'm guessing seeing her friends walking off with her mum and dad, made reality sink in. Her friends could go home and go out for the evening and she was stuck in here! Although Luke and John got on my nerves (and they were beginning to notice) I had to feel sorry for them. In the three weeks I was there (Three weeks! I feel such a wimp. There were people who had spent most of their lives sectioned in one way or another) I never saw them get any visitors but it was Ennio I had the most sympathy for. In a foreign country, in a foreign hospital, in a foreign nuthouse, can't speak the lingo and still just a kid with absolutely no one to visit him. No wonder he used to scream out at night!

Medication time.
Dominique finally gave in and took her meds (which went straight down the sink at the nearest opportunity) Me, Maz, Zee and Dominique were in the games room and I asked her why she kept singing that song. Big mistake! Out came a C.D and she told us all that it was a demo of a single she was hoping to get released. She went over to the stereo and turned off the Floyd (I wasn't happy) and stuck on what can only best be described as Jerry Halliwell with a hangover! It was bloody awful but none of us had the heart to tell her and we all said how great it was. She wasn't a bad person really, just a tad bit too sure of herself and

clearly had bipolar too. I could fully appreciate her feelings of grandeur as I felt exactly the same (I just displayed it in a different way)

I'm not too bad at art and used to draw these big pictures of various subjects. I knew that I wasn't that good really but with the bipolar, all it took was one person to say,"Wow, that's great!" and then I really started to believe it. When my brother Davey came to pick me up and take me back in to the hospital, I took one of my pictures with me because they had a bit of an art gallery thing going on and I thought it would be a good idea to add something to it. There was a reason behind my thinking also. This particular picture was called something like, '523 million, 221 thousand, 367 seconds, drawn by the millions and millions and millions of molecules of John Barrett'

It depicted my very first memory, up to the first time I ever met my wife and was one of those pictures you could spend ages looking at because it contained so many images. I thought it would be a good idea if the doctors could see it as they walked past the gallery and think to themselves, "Hmm, now what does this tell us about Mr. Barrett?"

That night and with no Lucy for company, I started talking to Dominique. She had seen my drawing on the wall and her first response was, "You must draw me!"

I told her that I'd do it tomorrow and then we sat at one of the dining tables and Amanda (head nurse that night) watched us from the nurse's station. By now, they had all given up telling us to go to bed. As long as we were quiet, they figured it would be simpler to just let us tire ourselves out and go to bed of our own accord. Zee, Maz and Luke came out of their rooms

SECTION 2: MEDIUM

and joined us. I can't remember why but the conversation steered to all things supernatural and I started joking that we should make one of those ouigee boards. Dominique got sharp with me and told me not to fuck about with things like that. I started to laugh but quickly noticed that everyone else agreed with her. We all then started to tell each other stories about weird things that had happened to us (it was like one of those 70's British horror films, where there are loads of short stories)
I started off and told them about the time I was in my flat on the same computer I am writing this now. It was about 3:30am and I was completely alone. Totally sober, typing something or other, when someone (or something!!!!!!!!!) touched me on the shoulder!

CHAPTER 26

I felt a finger pressing down firmly on my right shoulder and obviously being surprised, turned around to see who it was. There was no one there of course; the flat was completely empty apart from me. I did not think, "Fucking hell" or anything at all, I just accepted it and continued writing, totally believing someone had just touched me. As I was telling the others this, I was starting to get the creeps just thinking back on it and our surroundings didn't help either. Imagine being in a very large room, sitting at a round table with our backs a long way away from any of the walls, in very low light and screaming sounds coming from Sherrin below us. Maz told the rest of us that he had trouble sleeping and when he woke in the middle of the night, there would always be a young girl sitting at the end of his bed. She would be dressed in a nightgown and was soaking wet, as if she had drowned but she never spoke to him. Zee, Luke and Dominique all had similar experiences of either seeing or feeling the presence of a ghost. It was only some time after being discharged I began to think what a coincidence it was that we had all experienced something weird. I then came to the conclusion that when someone has suffered trauma in one way or another, their mind starts to play tricks on them. Maybe it is a cry for help or something but I fully believe it's all in that person's imagination. That night in my flat, I really did believe that someone touched me on the shoulder, I was completely convinced of it but the mind is a strange thing and I now think it was my mental state which made me believe it to be true. After all, the brain controls our feelings and so maybe it was telling me I felt that touch. Oh, I don't bleedin' know do I. That's my theory anyway and I'm sticking to it!

We eventually made our way back to our rooms. Zee was now sharing a bedroom with Chris and Luke and I had Derek and John Barnet either side of me. As soon as I went into our room, my nostrils were bombarded with the foul stench of very smelly feet. I knew it couldn't be Derek because he would always get up at about eight or nine at night and after a few coffee's, go and have a shower and then spend up to about three in the morning, styling his hair into the perfect quiff and so that only left John.
They were both obviously sound asleep because they were snoring like mad and so I turned the light on and pulled back the curtain surrounding John's bed. His feet were sticking out of the sheets and what can best be described as mushrooms were growing between his toes. I felt sick and pushed his back to wake him up. He just mumbled something and carried on snoring. I pushed him again, harder this time but he still didn't wake up. It was no use; he must have been drugged up to the eyeballs.
"Fuck it!"
I went to my bedside cabinet and got some aftershave out, dabbed some all around my nostrils and then got my deodorant and nearly emptied the can on his foul feet! I felt tired, sick and pissed off, all at the same time and got into bed and closed my eyes, trying to ignore the stench but couldn't go to sleep. That rank

odour overpowered all my attempts to defeat it (no pun intended)

It must have been about 4am and I was slipping in and out of conciencness. The curtains were pulled completely around my bed (it was the only way to get any privacy in that place)

Was I dreaming but did the door creak slowly open, followed by the sound of feet shuffling across the floor. Not much light, only the faint glow from the hallway outside.

Silence.............I must be dreaming.

Suddenly my curtains were pulled back and I saw Chris standing at the end of my bed, looking as white as a sheet.

"FUCK!" he scared the life out of me because it took a few seconds for my eyes to adjust in the dim light.

"Chris, what are you doing out of bed?" I asked.

He was mumbling something over and over so I got up and stood next to him, so I could hear better.

"Toilet, I need the toilet" he whispered.

"What a fucking night this has turned out to be," I thought and led him to the men's toilets, just off the hallway outside.

No sign of any staff around and so I took him into the toilet and started to pull down his pyjama bottoms. Right at that moment, Chris shit himself (big time) and I couldn't decide what was worse, his arse or John's plates of meat. I pulled his trousers down the rest of the way and sat him on the toilet.

"Wait there," I told him and went off in search of a staff member.

The nurse's station light was on but when I went up to the window, I could see there was no one there.

"FUCK, FUCK, FUCK!"

SECTION 2: MEDIUM

I went to the laundry room and got a spare pair of pyjamas and some towels and then made my way back to Chris. No contest in the Chris and John stench bout, Chris's arse won by a knockout. I tell you, that smell nearly did knock me out too! I was just about to clean him up when two female orderlies I'd never seen before, appeared in the doorway.

"What the hell do you think you're doing!" one of them asked me in a stern voice.

"You're fucking job!" I shouted and went back to my bed and the now, sweet smelling odour of John's feet.

CHAPTER 27

7am, 28th December.

I was woken by Davina the nurse entering our room. My curtains were still pulled back from the Chris incident and she said good morning. I replied with the same, got up and grabbed a towel and some shower gel.
"Who's in there?" she whispered, pointing to the curtain surrounding John's bed.
"Mr. Smelly"
"I fucking heard that, you bald headed cunt!" yelled John.
"Fuck you fat boy!" I replied while walking off to the shower room.
After my shower I returned to my bedroom and guessed that John must have gone for his breakfast because he wasn't in his bed but Derek was still fast asleep as usual. I splashed on some aftershave and put on my best whistle and just for a change, wore some comfortable black trainer type thingies and headed off for coffee and brekkies! Mo was on duty and he commented on how smart I looked but said the trainers let it down.
"One moment," I told him, "I'll fix that in a jiffy".
I walked back to the bedroom and changed into smart shoes, then went back to Mo. "Happy now?" I asked him.
"That's much better," he replied.

Victoria, the head nurse in charge (the one who I said was just like Nurse Ratched in Cuckoos Nest) was also on duty and she gave me a dirty look.
"Fuck me!" roared Zee as he walked into the hall, "Look at you!"
"I've got my review with the doctor," I explained, "and want to look the part"
"Nice one, now what shit we got to eat today?"
Dominique came out of the lady's wing and gave me a wolf whistle and John and Luke gave me the daggers while they ate their breakfast and whispered to each other. The young nurse who took me and Maria to have our blood tests, came out of the nurse's station and also said how smart I looked. Dominic and Craig sat with me and Zee, while Ennio sat with Chris and Maz.
"Lucy is back this morning," said Zee.
"I know. She was acting strange the last couple of days before going home"' I replied.
"You know why, don't you," said Zee and nodded his head in the direction of Dominique.
"That's what I thought; you don't think she is jealous do you?"
"Nah, she just doesn't like people who are loud and cocky. Did she tell you she was raped when she was a school girl?"
I nodded and took a bite of my jam on toast, deciding that it was probably best not to mention about Lucy's dad.

Me and Zee went for a fag (shadowed by the ashtray vultures) and there was this guy from the ward above ours. He asked me to meet him here at 6 o'clock tonight and he'd show me all the stars and their names.

I told him okay (I like all that stuff) and smoked another cigarette before making my way back up to our ward and by the time I reached the hall, it was time for my review.

"Good luck mate….I'll keep my fingers crossed!" said Zee and slapped me on the back, nearly knocking the wind out of me in the process.

Walking along the corridor past my room and opening the door leading to the assessment and review room, I stopped to look at my reflection in a window and readjusted my tie.

I then knocked loudly, three times on the door.

"Come in," said a muffled voice on the other side and so I entered the room and casually walked over to a leather couch and sat down opposite the doctor and Nelson.

They both looked at each other as I crossed my legs one over the other and placed both hands gently on my knees.

"You look very smart today John," said the doctor appearing somewhat surprised and coughed into his hand.

"So do you doc," I replied, coughing into my own hand and mimicking him exactly, "but not as smart as me eh," and then tapped the side of my head with my finger.

(Not the cleverest thing to do)

He smiled politely and then wrote something down on the clipboard resting on his lap.

My decision to take a couple of suits with me into the hospital when I was readmitted was solely because I wanted to take the piss but looking back at it now, I clearly wasn't taking my situation in the least bit seriously.

SECTION 2: MEDIUM

The doctor mentioned about my fast driving again, when I travelled down from my flat to Hampshire and I explained that I was perfectly in control of the car. I asked again if I could have a single bedroom because John's feet were making me feel sick.

"I'll tell you what I'll do doctor," I said, "you sleep next to him tonight and I'll go home to your bed"

He tried not to laugh and whispered something to Nelson, who then explained that they were 'full to capacity'

I just shrugged my shoulders, flicked a piece of fluff off my trouser leg and decided that I would sleep in the games room that night, on the massage chair (not switched on, I hasten to add!)

The doctor and Nelson talked in hushed tones for a while and then told me they didn't think I was ready to be discharged just yet and my next review would be on New Years Eve at 4 o'clock.

I wasn't in the least bit surprised and nodded my head, got to my feet and wished the doctor a good day.

Maria was sitting on a sofa by the entrance to the lady's wing when I entered the hall and I decided to join her. We were opposite the main door to our ward and I saw Stewart walk in with Lucy. He nodded a greeting to me and then gave her a hug, said a few words and left. She had a folder and scrapbook under her arm and was looking the happiest I had ever seen her.

"Hi Luce" I called out as she walked over and knelt down by the side of the sofa.

"Stewart got these from my mum," she explained and put the scrapbook and folder on my lap.

When I opened up the folder, it was full of old school reports and certificates for sports. All the reports said that she was a very keen student and worked very hard but was always quiet and didn't communicate much with the other pupils. I opened the scrapbook and there were loads of newspaper clippings of Lucy at running and swimming charity events.

"This is for you John," she said and gave me a pamphlet with a picture of a dove and a crucifix on the cover. I gazed down at it and she told me to look inside. Stewart had told her that she should write a little about herself and they could have it printed up for the next church meeting. It did not mention about the cab driver incident and certainly not what her dad did to her but told of her years in institutions and the time she found god and how he had given her strength.

"You're crying, aren't you," she whispered and put her hand on my arm.

I didn't say anything; I just got up and walked in the direction of the games room.

"What's the matter with him?" I heard Dominique ask Lucy.

"Nothing, leave him alone"

Zee was playing pool with Maz and could see I was upset.

"You wanna game next?" he asked.

Zee was trying to lift my spirits and knew just like every other patient, not to ask what was wrong. We all had our own problems and understood when it was the right or wrong time to give someone support. I think he let me win our game but I didn't care, I was feeling a lot better. Dominique came in and actually asked if I was okay!!!!

So….she was human after all.

SECTION 2: MEDIUM

After lunch, an art teacher came in and said that she was having a class in the ward upstairs. I'd heard that they had a proper pub pool table and so jumped at the offer. Nigel (the Barclays bank manager) Luke and Dominique came too and it was true, there was a pub pool table! I thought it best if I did a bit of the art class first and started doing a sketch of Nigel as he worked on his own picture. Dominique wrote her name in BIG letters and started to colour it in, while Luke drew something religious or anarchistic! The man who told me to meet him at 6 o'clock for a spot of stargazing walked in and I asked him if he wanted a game of pool. It was such a nice table and the balls rolled sweet, a little too sweet because he beat me!
"Best of three?"
"Why not?"
I won the second game and he won the third and so I shook his hand and told him that I would see him later. Walking back to the art class table, Nigel asked me if he could keep the sketch of him as he thought it was really good. I told him he could and he explained that he loved to make pottery as a hobby and would show me some photo's of his work when we got back to our own ward. As we were making our way downstairs, Dominique asked (told) me, "Draw me, draw me!" and I told her that I'd do it later and went for a fag.
When I got back, Nigel showed me his photos and they were beautiful. All different shaped vases and bowls, in bright vivid colours. I told him they were brilliant and had he sold any. He looked at me bashfully and said that his wife was looking into it. I reckon he knew they were good when he was of a

level frame of mind but now he was feeling low, all of his confidence had completely vanished.

Six o'clock arrived and I met the star man downstairs. He seemed like a nice bloke and we talked for a while before he started explaining which stars were which. I can only remember a few of them but the thing that really struck me was when he said, "Can you see those tiny, tiny stars?" and pointed to something barely visible.

I nodded and he continued, "Well, they aren't stars at all but satellites orbiting the earth"

That blew me away and I spent the next 10 minutes with my eyes fixed on the night sky. So next time it's a clear night, go outside and look very carefully, you might just see some moving slowly overhead.

After dinner and meds, it was visiting time and my mum and Pauline arrived but for some reason I was anti them and didn't want to talk much. I suppose I blamed them for me being sectioned but just for the record Paul, it was the best thing that ever happened to me. That experience has given me some understanding of my symptoms (although at the time, I didn't know it)

Please don't feel guilty about what happened and of course I know you did it for my best interests.

As soon as they left, I wanted them to come back. What was wrong with me?

They had travelled 130 miles to see me and I didn't even want to speak to them, I felt so bad. That night, Lucy, Zee (all suited up, with a pork pie hat) Maz, Dominic, Craig, Dominique and I played pool until lights out. I said that I was having an early night and went to my bedroom. John and Derek were asleep (come to think of it, I can't remember Derek being up

and about at all that day) and I smoked cigarettes out the window until I could hear all of the others go to bed. When they had all gone, I gathered up my blanket and pillow and crept back into the games room. I then threw the blanket over the massage chair, put down my pillow and climbed aboard the contraption.
"Ahhh......ABSOLUTE BLOODY BLISS!"
No smells, no snoring, just me on my own and at long last, a decent night's sleep!

"AAAAAAAARRRRRGGGGGHHHHHH!!!!!!!!!"
I was woken at about 2am by Dominique standing above me, shaking my shoulders and screaming at the top of her voice! Although dark, I could see it was Dominique and she wouldn't stop screaming. All of a sudden, the games room lights came on and one of the night shift nurses ran in.
"What's going on!" she shouted.
Dominique started laughing really loudly and said, "Just trying to liven this fucking place up!"
The nurse was clearly not in a good mood, "Why are you sleeping in here?" she asked me.
"You try getting to sleep with those stinking feet!" I replied.
She turned back to Dominique, "Right, you get back to your own bedroom.....NOW!"
"I'm gone bitch!" and with that, she strolled out of the games room and back to her own room, still laughing out loud all the while.
"John, I want you to go back to your room"
"No"
"Do you want me to call the orderlies up from downstairs?"

"Look, I'm not causing any trouble. I just want to get a decent night's sleep, that's all!"
She thought for a moment and then seemed to calm down.
"Well?......okay but don't let anyone else know about it" she said.
"Just keep your eyes open for that mad bitch"
"Goodnight John"
She closed the games room door quietly behind her and turned the lights off.
"Jesus Christ, will I ever have any time to myself?"
I went over to the window and had a cigarette and then went back to the chair and fell asleep.

CHAPTER 28

29th December, 6am

The lights came on and Luke walked in, obviously in a weird state. He was mumbling what I guessed were passages from the bible and his eyes were staring wildly ahead of him. He didn't notice me (the massage chair was in the corner) and walked over to the pool table and set the balls up. It was only as he was about to break that he saw me in his line of view.
"So.......it's the devil himself! What say we have a game of pool Satan? I'll be on the side of Jesus!"
I got out of the chair and got dressed, "Okay then, you play for Jesus and I'll play for myself"
"The anti-Christ!"
"Whatever. I'm gonna grab a coffee and go for a smoke first"
I saw the wild look soften briefly and then return to its feral gaze. The son of God could hardly ask Satan for a fag, now could he! As I made my way to the main door which led to the stairs leading down to the courtyard, I nodded to the night shift nurse who'd let me stay in the games room.
"Fuck it, I almost slipped up there!" I said to myself and quickly knocked on the nurse's station door.
"Can I have my cigarettes and lighter please"
I'd nearly gone outside with my own stash and that would have given the game away. She gave me my stuff and I went downstairs, thinking about the ensuing game of pool. After a couple of fags, I walked

back upstairs and noticed there was still no one else awake apart from Luke. I got a coffee from the vending machine and walked back to the games room where Luke was sitting in a chair with a cue across his lap, his eyes still staring wildly.

"You break" he told me in a monotone voice.

I picked up the other cue, leant down and broke. Jesus was out of his chair like a shot, scanning the table and then went for a yellow ball. I had never seen anyone strike so hard and not only that, the yellow found the perfect centre of the middle pocket.

The words, "Shit! I'm in trouble here!" raced through my mind and he repeated the process with the next two yellows but missed the pocket on the next shot. I managed to pot my first red but missed the second. Luckily, I left the cue ball safe. Jesus aimed his cue again and I could see the intense concentration on his face. Slam! He went for a pot and missed and split the remaining colours all over the table. My reds were in a great position and I potted the next two but left the cue ball in an awkward position. I needed to concentrate and took my time aiming the cue up to the white ball. Jesus knew I was in trouble and as I was about to take my shot he called out, "Evil will never conquer the goodness of Christ. God will keep my aim straight and true!"

I blanked him out and striked the cue ball. The red rolled slowly over to the middle pocket and only just went in, leaving me to clear up the remaining reds.

"Shit" I whispered.

The black ball was tight against the cushion and the white was up the other end of the table. I'm not good enough to get a safety shot from that position and so I just hoped for the best and went for it.

SECTION 2: MEDIUM

"Shit, shit!"
The black stopped roughly twelve inches away from the top corner pocket and the cue ball was perfectly in line about thirty inches away. Luke took his time on the shot and I noticed that he didn't hit it so hard this time. He missed the pocket and left the black on the white spot, while the cue ball ended up in the middle of the table. Once again, he started preaching all this stuff and so I decided to shut him up once and for all. I didn't take my time and just whacked the white ball, going for a double in the bottom corner. As the black bounced off the top cushion, I put my cue down and turned towards the games room door. The black went in; I know because Luke yelled, "Lucky cunt!"
Without turning around I said, "And it's John One, Jesus Nil"
I decided it was best if I went for another smoke and kept out of his way for a while, otherwise he might have turned me into a pillar of salt or something.

A strange thing happened at breakfast.
Luke walked over to me and shook my hand and was all friendly and even started talking sense! John was sitting on his own, eating his breakfast and I went over to him and apologised. He shook my hand too and also said sorry. Lucy was sitting on one of the sofas and was surrounded by all of her teddy bears and cuddlies which she usually kept on her bed. I went over to her and asked if she was okay. She seemed happy and calmly asked me to sit down next to her.
"Stewart is trying to get the doctors to let me go home with him for good!" she said.
"That's great Luce, Stewart is a really nice bloke!"

Lucy passed me a purple teddy bear and whispered, "This is for you. When I'm gone, he will remind you of me"
"Thanks Luce, that means a lot" I replied.
We both got up and stood in line for our meds and I noticed that even Dominique was queuing up! Back in the games room and I gave my tablet to John while Dominique gave hers to Luke (they weren't fussy about our saliva)
My cousin Lee visited me again and I asked Victoria if he could take me to my flat, so I could get a change of clothes. I couldn't believe it when she agreed but told Lee that he was responsible for me. Derek overheard the conversation and asked me if I could get him some Brylcream as he was running low. I told him I would then followed Lee to his car, got in and he floored it!

We reached my place in fifteen minutes flat and headed straight for the pub. Man, that first beer tasted good! When we went out the back for a smoke, the bargirl joined us. She asked me where I had been and I explained everything to her and when I got to the bit where I had a panic attack, she said that she was driving on the motorway once and had one as well.
Apparently, her ex was a real git to her and as a result, she was really messed up (everyone has their own problems)
After sinking a couple of more beers, we went to Sainsbury's to get Derek's hair gel. I bought him three tubs as I didn't know when he would have the chance to get some more and the girl behind the till gave me a funny look, obviously thinking, "Why does a bald headed bloke need hair gel?"

SECTION 2: MEDIUM

We then went back to the flat and while Lee grabbed himself another beer from the fridge, I went through the post. It was just boring stuff like credit card bills (I threw them to one side) but the last envelope made my day. I had copied an image off Google of a still from the film Vanishing Point, where the Dodge Challenger is being followed closely by a police helicopter. I sent it to Truprint's website and had an A4 size photo made up of it. That was going to take pride of place above my hospital bed! As I was upstairs getting some fresh clothes, Lee was playing around with my smart car in the car park.

When we arrived back at the hospital, Lee said that he had to get going and after seeing me back into my ward, made his way home. I handed over two packs of cigarettes to Tina (who had just come on duty) and stashed the other three. After unpacking my stuff and putting the picture above my bed, I walked into the hall and got a coffee. Dominique came out of the lady's wing and called out to me, "John, I've been looking all over for you!"
"They let me go home for a couple of hours"
"That's not fucking fair! How comes I can't go home?"
"You have to be assessed by the doctor first, it will probably be today or tomorrow," I replied.
"It's today. My mum and dad are coming for it, at 4 o'clock this afternoon. So it's possible I can get out of this place today?"
"If you behave yourself and be a good girl"
"Heh?"
"Yeh, it's possible" (no fucking way, I thought to myself)

"Wait there!" she said all excited and ran back to the lady's wing. I noticed Tina looking at me through the nurse's station window, so I gave her a wink and she returned the compliment. Zee and Maz were playing pool and seem happy enough, while Dominique returned with some scrapbooks under her arm and told me to sit down at one of the dining tables. She sat next to me and opened the first book. It was full of photos of her at drama school, dancing and singing on stage. I wasn't really interested but nodded my head anyway and said how good they were, just to be polite and more importantly, to keep her in a good mood. As she turned the pages, her arm brushed against mine and I felt goose bumps. The next book contained photos of girls pole-dancing in her studio and I asked her if she could do it.

"Easy!" she replied, "My body is very flexible!"

With that she stood up, lifted her right leg above her head and balanced on her left leg and I was glad I was sitting down, with my lower half under the table!

"That's brilliant!" I said, "You'll have to show me all your moves"

She put her leg down and came back to the table.

"If you get a couple of crash mats out of the games room, I'll show you my dance routine this afternoon!"

"Great!"

It was the first time I had ever seen her in a really good mood and I started to laugh.

"What's so funny?"

"Nothing.....it's just nice to see you happy!"

She grabbed my head and kissed me on the cheek, then got up, took her books and skipped off back to the lady's wing, calling out behind her, "I'll put my leotard on!"

SECTION 2: MEDIUM

"It's not so bad in here after all," I mused, "I'll let the rest of the boys know about this afternoon's performance!"

The news spread like wildfire and after lunch, Nigel (the suicidal bank manager) set some chairs out around the crash mats I'd laid down.

"So what time is she going to do her lap dancing, John?" he asked.

"It's not lap dancing Nige, its artistic dancing"

Zee, Maz, Craig, Nigel, Dominic, Ennio, myself and even a couple of guys from the upstairs ward, all sat around the crash mats and waited with baited breath. I turned around and noticed Victoria looking out the nurse's station window with a puzzled expression on her face. Just then, the lady's wing door burst open and out came Dominique in a very tight pink leotard. She squealed with delight at the sight of her audience and immediately went into her routine. Gord Blimey! I didn't know where to look! At one point, Dominique was on all fours in front of me, with her pink arse shoved in my face and her own face peering out from between her legs, upside down with black hair hanging down around it.

"Do you like it John?" she asked gleefully.

"Yeh, yeh!" I stammered, "It's, it's really good!"

I was like putty in her hands! Dominic looked at me and we both start grinning like little kids.

"Yeh baby!" yelled Zee and started clapping his hands together.

Nigel sat in silence, staring at the wonderful spectacle before him and a few of the other guys gave out wolf whistles. Suddenly, Ennio got up and rushed off to the men's toilets while Dominique continued with her marvellous moves. I noticed Mo leaning against a wall with his arms crossed and a big smile spread across his face. All of a sudden, Victoria stormed out of the nurse's station and yelled at Dominique, "WHAT DO YOU THINK YOU'RE DOING?"

"What's it look like?" I replied as Dominique carried on, oblivious to everyone and everything around her.

"Dominique, stop it at once!" she shouted.

"Why, what harm is she doing?" called out Dominic.

Victoria had to think for a moment.

"It's er......it's breaching health and safety regulations!" she replied.

We all burst out laughing and Dominique finally noticed Nurse Ratched.

"Those crash mats are obstructing a clear escape route to the fire exit!"

Dominique got herself up off the floor and also started to laugh.

"Okay bitch, I get the message," she said and walked back to the lady's wing with a thunderous applause following her.

"Mr. Arleigh! Get those men back to their own ward and get someone to put these crash mats back where they belong!"

Mo quickly unfolded his arms, pushed himself away from the wall and did what he was told.

CHAPTER 29

After all the guys dispersed, me and Zee went outside for a smoke and couldn't stop laughing at what had just happened.

"You could see everything!" said Zee and I noticed some of the guys in the caged in area of the Sherrin courtyard, almost drooling at the mouth.

Zee gave his last bit of cigarette to John and said that he was going back inside, "It's fucking freezing out here!" he accurately observed.

"I'll just have one more for luck," I told him and gave the rest of the one I was smoking to Luke.

As I lit a new cigarette, I looked at the security fence housing the Sherrin patients. It was about eight feet high and angled inwards at the top, with barbed wire running around the edge. The orderlies walked in and out of the building from time to time and didn't seem to pay much attention. It was then that I realised I could get out of there in ten seconds flat! (Just watch Cuckoo's Nest)

Once anyone made it into our courtyard, all they had to do was go to the end of the garden and jump over the fence or just open the gate as it was usually unlocked. There were CCTV cameras everywhere but if you were quick, you could make it out of there.

From that moment on, I decided not to piss off any of the Sherrin guys because if they figured out how to climb the fence too, they could come and murder me in my sleep! I thought I'd give my sister Pauline a ring and went up the steps leading to the garden, so I was out of earshot of John and Luke and a few of the other guys from the upstairs ward. My brother-in-law Dave answered and sounded concerned about my well being. I can't remember what I started rattling on about but I must have been talking for about forty minutes and he listened patiently for all of that time. I don't think I even got to talk to Pauline (she must have been in a right state, poor thing) and when I hung up, I made my way back to the games room.

Luke had a Coldplay album on the stereo and the track playing was Viva La Vida. I wasn't a massive fan and so the song was starting to get on my nerves.
From that moment on until I was discharged, he would play it at every opportunity and it obviously got into my system because now, I absolutely love it and every time it's played, I get goose bumps all over and am right there back in that ward. I decided to leave the games room and found Lucy sitting down on one of the sofas.
"What have you done with the teddy bear I gave you," she asked me.
"I've got him sitting on my bed"
"That's good John, he'll look after you. I can't wait to go home with Stewart!"
"Is it definite then?"
"I think so, I'll know for sure tomorrow. Stewart is coming in with me to see the doctor for my review"
"I'll keep my fingers crossed for you"
We spent the rest of the night talking about this and that, while Dominique played pool with Maz and Zee.

SECTION 2: MEDIUM

11pm, lights out.
The guys in the games room all went off to bed (even Dominique, blimey!)
I was feeling tired myself (it must have been the beers I had earlier in the day) and told Lisa I was going to bed. She said she was too and made her way back to the lady's wing. As before, I went to my bed and grabbed the blanket and pillow but unlike before, teddy came too this time and then I got comfy in the massage chair. It took me a long time to get off to sleep, probably due to the fact that I kept thinking about Dominique's performance earlier in the day.
It was about 3am and I was in that half awake, half asleep state. In a semiconscious haze, I heard the games room door creak slowly open and I kept my eyes ever so slightly open. I could just about make out the head of the night duty nurse, peering in from the doorway and I heard her laugh under her breath at the sight of me cuddling the teddy bear. It must have been about six when I finally fell into a deep sleep and dreamt a vivid dream that seemed so real..........

I was lying on my bed next to John and Derek, staring up at the ceiling. It was the middle of the night and yet something told me that I had to get out of bed. As soon as I stood up, it was like there was a massive weight pressing down on my shoulders and I fell to the floor on my hands and knees. I could feel the pressure pushing against my back and peered over to the open door of our bedroom. I started to slowly crawl to the doorway and as soon as I got out into the corridor, the weight suddenly lifted but for some reason, I continued to crawl on my hands and knees. The corridor in the men's wing was divided up into a series of interconnecting fire doors, which were always shut at night but on this particular occasion, each one was still open and I could just about see through the dimness, right the way into the main hall. I made my way slowly along the corridor and upon reaching the hall, looked over to the nurse's station and to my surprise, all the lights were off. There weren't any members of staff on duty and no patients up either; I was all alone. Still crawling, I edge towards the lady's wing and in my head I could hear a voice calling me. As in the men's corridor, all of the fire doors were open and it was very dark but there was a full moon outside and it offered just enough light shining through the windows, to enable me to see where I was going. To my right, I passed the medicine room and to my left, Maria and Ann's room.

The voice was getting louder and when I reached the next open doorway on the left, I could see Dominique sitting on the edge of her bed (in reality, she shared with Maria and Ann)

"Come over here John," she whispered and so I crawled over to her and rested my head on her lap. She placed the flat of her hand on top of my head and told me to stand up and as I did so, she got to her feet as well. I placed my hand around the back of her head and pulled her closely towards me and we started to kiss. Dominique then very gently took my hand away and grabbed hold of the other before pulling me down on the bed and then....................

SHIT!

Davina marched into the games room and shouted that breakfast was being served!

CHAPTER 30

7am, 30th December.

Even though I'd hardly had any sleep, I was feeling as right as rain and took my blanket and pillow and teddy back to my bed and had a full head shave before taking a shower. I started singing Dead Flowers by the Stones; at the top of my voice (I love that song!)
Back in my bedroom and Derek was snoring as usual but John was actually awake (he must have smelt the breakfast cooking)
"Morning John," I said.
"Morning John," he replied.
I was feeling good and on a high and so decided to wear my favourite suit.
John asked me if he could listen to some of my Pink Floyd CD's on his Walkman and I told him to help himself, then walked into the main hall with the dream about Dominique still in my mind. There was no sign of Maz but Zee was sitting with Dominic, Craig and Ennio. All of a sudden, Dominique came marching in and was obviously in a bad mood. She was effing and blinding at anything that moved and I was immediately turned off by her.
She then went over to the nurse's station and started banging on the glass.
"I want to see that useless fucking doctor, right now!"
Lucy walked into the hall and I asked her what was wrong with Dominique.

"She had her review yesterday afternoon and it didn't go the way she wanted"
"But I saw her playing pool last night and she seemed okay?"
"Zee said she was really quiet, it obviously didn't sink in until this morning"
"Great, so we've got another fucking day of her ranting and raving"
"Looks like it," replied Lucy and went off to get her breakfast.
Mo came out of the nurse's station and tried to calm Dominique down.
"Your next review is in three days' time, the doctor explained that to you yesterday"
"Fuck you fatso!"
"Just calm down and have something to eat"
"What, that fucking shit!"
I know I shouldn't have but I felt I had to say something. "Do everyone a favour and shut the fuck up you spoilt little brat!"
"Go fuck yourself baldy and who the fuck do you think you are in that fucking suit, God or something?" (She'd obviously spent some time with Luke)
"I'm crazy Dominique, just like you!"
"I ain't nothing like you loony fuckers!"
Mo was then joined by Davina and they stepped closer to Dominique, "If you don't sit down now, I will send for a doctor and it won't be for the reason you're hoping for!" he explained to her.
"I told you fatty, fuck off!"
Mo turned to Davina and nodded and then she went back into the nurse's station and picked up the phone.
"You stupid cow," I thought to myself, "when are you going to learn?"

SECTION 2: MEDIUM

Two orderlies and a senior nurse arrived on the scene and dragged Dominique back to the lady's wing, accompanied by the usual expletives!

Lucy's review was at 11am.
Stewart arrived at 10:30 and he and Lucy walked into the quiet room, where I was sitting.
"Do you want me to leave?" I asked them.
"No, no, not at all," replied Stewart.
They both sat down opposite me and Stewart once again tried to bestow his beliefs on me. I told him that I respected his beliefs but not to preach them to me because I wasn't interested. I explained that I was always polite to people and didn't swear in everyday conversations and was always courteous.
"That's the way I was brought up and without a hint of God in sight"
Stewart laughed and said that one day I'd understand and then he and Lucy got up and went for her review.
I had left one of my DVD's by the T.V and noticed Ennio reading the back of the box.
Had he been fooling us all along and could actually understand English after all?
After about half an hour, Lucy and Stewart came out of the review and I could see she was low.
"How'd it go?" I asked Stewart.
He seemed quite positive, "The doctor says that Lucy has improved greatly but feels that she still needs to be monitored but hopefully she will be discharged on her next review"
I knew not to touch Lucy on the shoulder and simply said that she only had to wait three more days. She looked at the ground and nodded her head slightly. I

then felt it was best to leave them alone and decided to go for a smoke (any excuse)
The rest of the day was filled up with a marathon pool tournament which included me, Zee, Maz, Craig, Dominic and sometimes Lucy. There was no sign of Dominique (obviously drugged up and out for the count)

After dinner and meds, visitors started to enter the main hall. Maz's mum and dad arrived and they were sitting over by the T.V. Sarah (Myra Hindley) had with her, who I presumed to be her brother or sister and their partner and they were sat close to Maz. Chris's long suffering wife sat with him at a dining table while me and Zee sat at another. Craig's parents were allowed to go into his private room and talk to him there, while Dominic went out for an hour to see his girlfriend. Lucy must have been asleep because I couldn't see her anywhere and Maria sat on a sofa with her mother and sister (who looked just like her) or how she would have looked if she hadn't lost her marbles.
Dominique appeared out of the lady's wing and looked all sheepish. She got a coffee and sat down with me and Zee. The three of us sat there in silence and watched the other patients with their relations. Lots of staff were on duty and they were all in the nurse's station, laughing and joking about something or other. All of a sudden, Sarah stood up and then went into a trance like state and fell over. She dropped like a dead weight and didn't even use her hands to break her fall, hitting her head on the side of the T.V cabinet as she did so. Maz's dad immediately got up to help her.

SECTION 2: MEDIUM

"Oi in there!" yelled Zee, "Sarah's fallen over!"
The staff all looked up and Dominique was pointing over to where Sarah lay on the floor. Nurse Ratched walked briskly out of the nurse's station and had to pass our table to get to Sarah.
"<u>You</u> lot should be dealing with this, not the visitors!" I told her sternly.
She said nothing but looked at me irritably and then made her way over to Sarah. Her head was smothered in blood and Nurse Ratched knelt down to examine her before calling out to Victor and another male nurse to get a stretcher trolley and once they had returned, they wheeled her off to casualty in the main hospital. I looked at Maz's parents and they both had concerned expressions on their faces as if to say, "Is our son safe here?"

Dominique's mum and dad and one of her friends arrived shortly after and she introduced me to them. I got on really well with them and Dominique told her friend that I was a bit of a film buff. She asked me what type of movies I liked and I said that was impossible to answer because there were too many! I could see Zee through the window of the games room, playing pool on his own and felt so sorry for him. He desperately wanted to see his wife and son but it just wasn't going to happen until he learnt to control his violent temper and I honestly didn't know if he could. Dominique's dad looked fidgety and was playing with a tin of cigars. I told him where the smoking area was outside and joined him for a cigarette. He explained to me about Dominique's erratic behaviour and I could recognise myself immediately. It's funny, everyone was telling me I had bipolar and I refused to accept it but when someone explained the classic symptoms of another sufferer, I recognised it straight away. I think it was at that point that I started to believe I had the condition myself.

When we finally went back upstairs, Dominique's dad gave me two of his cigars and I decided that I would give one of them to Zee and we could smoke them the following night (and what a night that turned out to be!)

CHAPTER 31

All of the visitors had left and Maz was looking a bit low (I guess he was missing his mum and dad) and he went off to his room. I pointed it out to Davina and she said that she'd keep an eye on him. Tina was on duty that evening and was sitting outside Ennio's, doing the suicide watch. I walked up to her and asked if she wanted a cup of coffee.

"Not at the moment John but I'll have one when someone takes over from my watch at nine"

"Then it's a date, I'll meet you at nine by the vending machine and buy you a free cup of coffee!" I replied and as I walked back down the corridor to the main hall, I could hear her laughing to herself. Davina came out of one of the men's rooms with some dirty laundry (probably Chris's) and looked at me and then down the corridor, towards Tina. She turned back to me and had a suspicious expression on her face.

"Evening," I said and carried on walking to the main hall. There wasn't any sign of Lucy (she must have been in her room) and John and Luke were sitting at one of the dining tables, talking among themselves.

Looking through the games room doorway, I could see Dominique and Zee playing pool. They called out to me to join them but I wasn't really in the mood and went to the nurse's station to ask for a couple of cigarettes.

Outside and there was this lady I'm guessing was in her mid sixties but it was hard to tell. She was with the star gazer guy from upstairs and they had an orderly

with them. I noticed she was smoking a roll up and was down to about the last quarter of an inch. Her fingers were almost black with nicotine stains and she was shaking all over (although that could have been to do with the cold, it was fucking freezing!)
She told me that she'd been admitted about a month earlier after having a breakdown when her house had burned down. The star gazer man put his arm around her and whispered that everything would be alright in the end. It turned out that she was from the same village as me and I felt really sorry for her. She must have been burning her fingers with her roll up and so I gave her my other cigarette. The orderly rummaged in his pocket and brought out a lighter and lit the cigarette for her and it was then that I realised what must have happened. Either by accident or on purpose, she'd obviously set light to her house and so couldn't be trusted to light up her own cigarettes. I patted her on the shoulder and said that I'd probably see her later and then made my way back inside.

Once inside the hall, I got myself a coffee from the vending machine and sat down with Luke and John. The "Mr. Smelly" remark I'd called John, must have had an impact because he looked clean and he'd obviously had a shower and so I decided to sleep back in my bed that night. We started talking about Pink Floyd and he knew all the makes of synthesisers that Rick Wright would use and started going on about different chords and stuff (he'd lost me at that point)
We must have looked pretty odd sitting there, three blokes with shaved heads, although John's hairdressing skills leaved a lot to be desired.

He had naturally, thick dark hair and there were clumps of it randomly spaced all over the back of his head. I didn't have the heart to tell him but offered to shave it again for him, the next time he wanted it done. During our pool marathon earlier in the day, I'd been playing 'Mind Bomb' by the group 'The The' and Luke commented on how much he'd liked it.

I told him that once we were discharged, I'd do a copy for him and send it to him if he gave me his address. He just looked down at the table and said nothing and I realised that he had nowhere to go to (I really felt sorry for him and quickly changed the subject)

"Have you always been religious Luke?" I asked and immediately wished I'd kept my bleedin' mouth shut!

"The others weren't into Jesus until I tried to show them the error of their ways," he replied.

"What others?"

"In the squat I lived in. They smoked dope all day long and took heroin all of the time. I never got into that, just a bit of smack every now and then until I found Jesus and he told me I had to stop and tell the others what he was telling me. At night, he would speak to me and say they had sinned but could still be saved!"

"Okay?" came my muted response.

I noticed that John looked down at the floor as I was speaking to Luke and seemed to be deep in thought.

"They blamed Blair and his government for all of our problems and I told them that they could solve everything by following the preaching's of the bible"

"What happened then?" I asked.

"They threw me out and so I got drunk and the next thing I remember, I was in this place"

He then got up and walked over to the vending machine for a coffee.

"My dad's coming to see me tomorrow night," said John.

"That's great, I bet you can't wait," I replied.

"He's bringing my headphones with him, the one's we got when I ended up in Sherrin. I'll be able to listen to you're Pink Floyd albums on them!"

"What headphones?"

"They cost £500 and are fucking awesome!"

"FIVE HUNDRED QUID!" I gasped, "For that money, they wanna be fuckin' awesome!"

"We were driving back home after getting them and a policeman pulled my dad over for something or other. I was still wearing the headphones when we got out of the car and while the policeman was talking to us, his walkie talkie started crackling and voices were coming out of it"

"Was it another copper talking to him?"

"It was at first but then another voice came on and it told me to look up in the sky"

"Eh?"

"I could hear it….the voice through my headphones"

"Oh right, of course," I replied in bemusement.

"Yeah and when I looked up, I could see this silver spaceship flying through the clouds!"

"What did he say then?" I said, thinking to myself that I was surrounded by total nutters but then again, I was in a fucking nuthouse so what did I expect! I was starting to accept that I'd had some sort of breakdown but these people had completely lost the plot!

"He said his people had designed my headphones and would communicate with me through them and then he told me to kill the policeman"

SECTION 2: MEDIUM

"What happened next?" I asked eagerly (This was getting interesting!)
"The policeman pinned me to the ground and in the struggle, the headphones fell off!"
"Why did he pin you to the ground?"
"I tried to attack him"
"Did you tell anyone about your special headphones?"
"The man in the spaceship said it was a secret and not to tell anyone. When my dad brings them in tomorrow, I can communicate with him again!"
Mo seemed to be the nurse who John got on with the most and I made a mental note to tell him in the morning.
"Don't let his dad bring those fucking headphones in!" For all I knew, E.T. might tell him to kill all of us too and he'll slaughter the lot of us in our beds! Luke returned with his cup of coffee and was mumbling something about Jesus forgiving the sinners, while John became quiet and withdrawn again. Derek came out of the men's wing (he'd obviously only just woken up) dressed in his usual robe and slippers and went and got himself a cup of tea. As he walked past I said, "Morning Derek!" but I don't think he got the joke.

CHAPTER 32

8:30pm and Ennio walked in listening to my iPod. He'd become completely attached to it and at one point I considered letting him keep it but had second thoughts; I love my music too much! He was followed into the hall by Tina, who looked over at me and smiled. She was carrying a clipboard and when she walked into the nurse's station, she placed it on the desk and started looking at it with Victor. He appeared to be asking her some questions and every now and then, she looked up and stared at me through the window. I went over to the vending machine to grab a coffee and stood behind Dominic who was getting a cup of tea.

"Alright John," he said, "how's it going?"

"I think Tina fancies me. I'm gonna ask her out on a date"

He turned around and looked at me in amazement.

"You're fucking mad mate, you can't ask a member of staff out!"

"Course I can. Like you said, I'm fucking mad remember"

"Seriously mate, don't go fucking about with Tina. I like her a lot and wouldn't want to see her upset!"

"Don't worry Dominic; I'd never do anything to hurt her"

With that, he leant in close and whispered, "You crafty little fucker!" and gave me a joke punch on the arm. Tina came out of the nurse's station, still carrying the clipboard and sat on the sofa nearest the exit,

opposite Ennio who was sitting over by the T.V. Dominic gave me a wink and walked off in the direction of the games room while Derek went back to our room (all the exertion of getting himself a cup of tea had worn the poor sod out!)
I'm making a joke of it but he really was very ill and it was touch and go if he'd make it to the rest of the week. It was his own doing really and I don't mean the alcohol but the fact that he refused outright to have a liver transplant. I made another coffee, walked over to the sofa and sat down next to Tina.
"How's John?" she asked.
"All the better for seeing you"
Davina was with Victor in the nurse's station and she kept staring at us when he wasn't looking.
"Are you happily married?" I whispered out the corner of my mouth, while staring down at Tina's wedding ring.
"The only happy part of my marriage is my kids," she whispered back.
"How many have you got?"
"Two girls and a boy. The eldest is twenty one and lives with her boyfriend and my second daughter is eighteen and lives at home with her ten year old brother"
"Do you live very far from here?" I asked whilst keeping an eye on Davina, keeping an eye on us.
"It's only a ten minute walk away and if I could do any more overtime, I would; just so I could get out of the house"
"What's the situation with Davina? What's with her staring at us?"
"We're friends outside of work and I think she can tell something is going on" she replied.

"Is something going on?"
Tina lifted the clipboard so it was in front of our laps and held my hand.
I looked at Davina through the nurse's station window and said to Tina, "Would you like to see me, when I get out of this place?"
"Yes"
Davina said something to Victor and then came out of the nurse's station and walked over to where we were sitting. Our hands parted at the last second as Davina leant down and asked if there was anything to report on Ennio. I stood up and told both Tina and Davina that I was going to play some pool. As I walked towards the games room, I turned around and saw them both staring at me.
"Shit!" I thought to myself, "I hope she doesn't say anything to that nosy cow, it could fuck up my review tomorrow!"

"Where the fuck have you been?" asked Dominique as she lay in the massage chair.
Dominic looked up from taking his shot on the pool table and smirked.
"Just talking to John and Luke out in the hall" I replied.
"What d'ya wanna talk to those two fags for?"
"I dunno….. just wanted a change of scenery I suppose"
Dominic took his shot and doubled the yellow ball off the top cushion into the bottom corner pocket.
"Shot my son!" barked Zee and slammed the butt of his cue on the floor.
I wandered over to Craig and watched him play on his Xbox for a while.

SECTION 2: MEDIUM

Dominique climbed out of the massage chair and propped herself up on the desk next to us.
"When are you going to draw my portrait then, John?"
"Tomorrow night," I lied, knowing that it was more than likely I'd be discharged by then.
"Why not do it now?"
"Nah, I'm knackered. I'm going to bed. Night everyone"
"Night son, see you in the morning," said Zee.
As I left the games room, Dominique called out, "Don't forget tomorrow night!"
"Yeah, yeah"
Derek was sitting on the end of his bed, listening to some rock and roll on his stereo. I went over to my bed and crouched down on the floor to get my cigarettes from under the bedside cabinet. I only just stood up in time when John walked in.
"That was close," I thought. "If he'd have seen where I stashed them, then he would have helped himself when I wasn't around"
I walked over to the window and opened it as far as it would go and offered John a cigarette which he accepted with gusto. Derek stood up and asked me if he could have one.
"I don't think you should mate," I told him, "It's not gonna do you any good"
"I don't give a fuck any more" he said in a low flat voice.
I gave him a cigarette and the three of us stared out of the window, smoking our lungs out while listening to Little Richard on the stereo.
Through the darkness of the window pane, tiny specks of bright orange light fell from the sky and then flames fluttered past.

"What the fuck is going on?" I asked, "It's raining fire!"
John looked at me and laughed, "It's that prick upstairs, setting light to stuff again"
Mental note: "Tell Mo in the morning, to move that lunatic to another room"
There was no way I wanted an arsonist above my bed!
I flicked the butt of my fag out of the gap in the window and told the others that I was going to bed.
"I'll turn the music down," replied Derek.
"That's alright mate, I like listening to music in bed; it helps me get off to sleep"
I pulled the curtain around me, stashed the cigarettes and lighter, got undressed and climbed into bed. John said goodnight to Derrick and then went to bed himself. I closed my eyes and couldn't wait for my review tomorrow afternoon; I just knew the doctor would discharge me this time!

CHAPTER 33

New Years Eve 2008.

The novelty of this place had worn off to say the least and I desperately wanted the doctor to discharge me when I had my review at 4pm. It was New Year's Eve for fuck's sake and I wanted to be down the pub that night! After my shower and shave, I decided not to wear a suit (I thought it best to stop taking the piss out of the doctors as this would only go against me in my review) and so wore jeans and a smart top. I had a strong feeling that I would definitely be discharged and the doctor had even given indications towards that direction in my previous review. I was in a good mood.

Both Nigel and Ann were due for their reviews at 11am and I wished them both good luck. Although I wasn't exactly the best of friends with Ann, I wouldn't have wished that place on anyone (unless they were dangerous) and she thanked me.

Lucy sat with me at breakfast and asked if I was nervous about my review.

"I am," I replied, "but also pretty confident at the same time"

"I think they'll discharge you John, I can feel it."

I looked over to Zee who was sitting with Chris and Sarah and he nodded but said nothing. I might have been wrong but I had the impression he was feeling slightly envious (if that's the right word) that it was looking very likely I was going to be discharged that

afternoon. Maz was nowhere to be seen and so after breakfast, I went to his room to check on him. He was sound asleep and one of the nurses popped her head round the door and said that she had tried to wake him for breakfast but he'd just shrugged and told her he didn't want any.
"See if you can wake him up," she told me and walked off down the corridor.
"Maz, Maz…..wake up mate, it's John"
I put my hand on his shoulder and shook him gently. He mumbled something in his sleep, which I couldn't make out.
"Come on Maz, its New Year's Eve. You don't wanna spend all day in bed like Derek"
"Get my clothes out of the wardrobe," he yawned and turned over onto his back.
I got up, went over to the cupboard and opened the door. There must have been twenty bottles of roll-on deodorant at the base of the wardrobe.
"Fucking hell Maz, what's with all the roll-ons?"
He took a great big yawn and said it was an obsessive thing he'd had for years.
"Well at least you smell nice!" I said and threw him his clothes. "Now get up, you lazy fucker"

I went outside for a cigarette and Mo was there, watching over Luke and John who'd managed to ponce a couple of fags off someone. It was a really sunny day, with not a cloud in the sky but absolutely freezing! Mo was really anti smoking and started telling me about the damage it was doing to my body.
"I know all that stuff, I'm addicted to it………it's a drug!" I explained.

"So you know full well that you're causing harm to your body and yet you still carry on doing it because you're addicted?" he replied.

"That's right," I said, patting his stomach, "just like you're addicted to food!"

"Come on you two, you've finished your cigarettes. Let's get back inside, it's freezing cold!" he called out, trying to change the subject. John and Luke were going through the bin as usual, looking for dog ends.

"Ah, the glamour of smoking," said Mo as I sparked up another.

"Inside now, both of you!" and off they went, with John staring longingly at my cigarette. When I got back upstairs, Dominique was standing by the entrance to the nurse's station. She seemed in a good mood and was chatting to Nelson and Mo about the cruise she should have been on.

"Morning," she said to me as I walked past. "Fucking hell, you stink of smoke. It's a horrible habit!"

"Don't you start, I've just had Mo on my case about that".

"What time is your review?" she asked.

"Four o'clock. By this time tonight, I should be down the pub sinking a few beers!"

I saw her face change and she looked down at the ground.

"Don't worry mate," I said, putting a hand on her shoulder," You'll be out of here soon"

We walked away from the nurse's station and over towards the games room.

"There's something wrong with me," she whispered.

I couldn't answer her because I was feeling exactly the same way about myself and it scared me. Finally I said to her, "I'll do a sketch of you after lunch if you like?"

That seemed to do the trick and she started to smile again.
"Great! I'll get out of my P.J's and put something nice on!" and with that, she walked off in the direction of the lady's wing.

Derek was up and dressed and it was only eleven in the morning, what was going on? He stood over by the vending machine and there was a man sitting at one of the dining tables, nearest to him. I walked over to the vending machine and asked, "You're up early Derek, what's the occasion?"
He looked at me with bleary eyes and nodded in the direction of the man sitting down.
"That's my brother Mark," he replied.
I could see the resemblance, they were both very similar except that Mark didn't have the greased back quiff or glasses. He got up and shook my hand.
"Alright mate," he said in a thick cockney accent. Derek walked away and sat down on one of the sofas by the T.V looking very depressed.
"Is everything okay?" I asked his brother, who didn't look too happy either.
"He's finally agreed to have a liver transplant and we've got an appointment this morning at this other hospital, to see the specialist"
"That's great!" I replied.
"He doesn't wanna fucking go now, the stupid cunt! Oi Derek, come on! Dad's waiting in the car, we're gonna be late!"
Derek rose to his feet slowly, put his plastic cup on a table and slouched off with his brother, to the main exit. I would have said good luck but somehow, it didn't seem to be appropriate. Both Nigel and Ann

came out from their reviews at the same time. Ann appeared to be very pleased with herself but Nigel didn't look too happy.

"How'd it go Nige?" I asked, expecting to hear a negative response.

"I've been discharged and my wife is coming to pick me up in an hour," he replied in a flat tone.

"Well that's good, innit?"

"Yes, I suppose so," he said and walked away. I could hear Ann telling Lucy that she'd been discharged also and walked over to her.

"What's wrong with Nigel?" I asked.

"He doesn't feel ready to leave yet but the doctors have convinced him that it's for the best"

I just shook my head and walked away, still not fully understanding how anyone would want to stay here.

"Can I have one of my fags Mo?" I asked, sticking my head round the door to the nurse's station. He shook his head slowly, went over to a drawer and pulled out about four different packs, looking for the one with my name on it. When he finally found the right one, he opened it up and began to laugh, "It's your last one, looks like you will have to give up after all"

"Oh shit! Look Mo, can I go over to the petrol station and get some more?"

I had two other packs stashed but couldn't let him know that. He thought for a moment and then said he would have a word with Victoria (Nurse Ratched) when she came in at twelve. That was only ten minutes away and I figured I could last out until then. I took my last cigarette, went downstairs and found Zee talking to one of the Sherrin orderlies through the wire fence. They were in a deep conversation and didn't notice me, so I went up to the garden and strolled around while I smoked. In one of the bins, I could see some empty beer cans and decided that if I was allowed to go to the petrol station, I'd get some for me and Zee to drink while we smoked the cigars Dominique's dad had given me. My original plan was to smoke them that night, to celebrate the New Year but seeing as it was looking more than likely I was going to be discharged following my review, I thought we could have them after lunch. When I returned to the ward, Victoria had come on duty and I stared at Mo through the nurse's station window, with a look that said, "Don't forget to ask her"

After about ten minutes, she called me in and explained that I could go but had to get back straight away. She then gave me £10 out of my money and I had another £10 in my sock.

"Remember John, get back here as soon as you've bought them" she reminded me.

I promised I would, then thanked her and made my way to the main reception area, where the double doors were, leading to the front car park. Derek's brother Mark was standing by the doors and was talking on his mobile phone.

"I don't fucking know do I. He said he had to go to the toilet and then fucking disappeared!" he said.

After hanging up, he looked at me and shook his head.

"What's happened?" I asked.

"The stupid cunt has done a runner! I knew this would happen, my old man is doing his fuckin' nut!"

"Why doesn't he want the operation?"

"I don't fucking know, he's scared or something and would rather fuckin' die. The stupid prick!"

SECTION 2: MEDIUM

Just at that moment, Derek walked through the entrance with his dad and they were both arguing with each other.
"Fucking leave me alone dad, I wanna go back to bed!"
"I don't know what we're gonna do with 'im Mark, we can't drag 'im there!"
Victoria and Nelson came through the doorway leading to our ward and she looked over at me.
"Haven't you gone yet John? Leave us to deal with this, now off you go"

It was only a five minute walk to the petrol station and when I got there, Davina was filling her car up with petrol.
"Shit!" I thought to myself, "That's the booze idea out of the window!"
She spotted me as I got to the forecourt and gave me a quizzical look.
"John, what are you doing?" she called out.
"Victoria said I could get some cigarettes. Don't worry; I'm going straight back again"
She nodded her head and carried on filling her car.
When I got back, I handed over my cigarettes to Mo and went to get a cup of coffee. I generally prefer tea but the stuff in the vending machine, tasted awful. Zee was playing pool with Maz and Dominic, while Craig was on his Xbox as usual. After lunch and meds, me and Zee went downstairs for a smoke and he couldn't believe it when I got out the cigars. Luke and John were there as usual, scavenging for dog ends and they looked on in disbelief as we puffed away, blowing out the blue/grey smoke in an exaggerated fashion. Mo shook his head but said nothing.

"Only two hours until your review mate," said Zee and blew out a perfect smoke ring.
"I can't wait; Melanie is coming in with me for support. She's really confident they'll discharge me!"
"Good luck son," he replied and stared off into the sky while rolling the cigar between his fingers. I noticed Mo staring at me with a serious expression on his face and wondered what was wrong with him. Back upstairs, I went to my room and stashed the tenner I still had in my sock, with the two packs of cigarettes under my bedside cabinet. I could hear talking coming from behind the curtains surrounding Derek's bed and recognised Melanie's voice but she was whispering and I couldn't make out what was being said. Lucy was sitting by the television with one of her teddy bears when I walked back into the hall and was looking sad. I decided not to approach her as I could tell she didn't want any company. When she'd told me the other day that she might get discharged, I was of course happy for her but at the same time, slightly jealous and I think she was feeling the same way now. Both Nigel and Ann had been discharged and it was looking almost certain that I would be too; she must have felt so depressed that she hadn't been.

I got myself another coffee (there was fuck all else to do, except drink coffee, smoke and play pool)
Maria was sitting with Davina whose shift had just started after she'd been at the petrol station. I sat down at one of the dining tables and stared at the clock on the wall, waiting for four o'clock. One hour to go. Sarah walked into the hall from the lady's wing, with a bandage wrapped round the top of her head. She seemed okay after the fall she'd had and went and sat

down on a sofa, next to the Christmas tree. Half an hour to go. Melanie came out from the men's wing looking upset and asked me if I'd like to join her for a cigarette, before we went in for the review. We walked downstairs and she burst out crying. It was the first time I'd ever seen her like that (she was usually such a tough person) and I put my arm around her shoulders to comfort her.

"He's going to die," she sobbed, "I don't think he'll even make it 'til the rest of the day!"

"Why is he doing this to himself?" I asked.

"I don't know but I've never spoken to someone who is so close to death before and they actually want to die. His skin is grey and he doesn't look like Derek anymore!"

A patient from the upstairs ward came outside for a smoke and Melanie pulled herself together and lit up a cigarette before offering me one. Putting on a brave face, she patted me on the arm and said, "Well John, are you ready for your review?"

I nodded and smiled but the news of Derek had put a bit of a dampener on my good mood. Melanie could sense this and whispered, "I'm sorry John, I shouldn't have put that on you. You've got yourself to worry about. Come on, let's go and see the doctor!"

I can't actually remember any of the review except the end, when the doctor told me that I wasn't ready to be discharged just yet and he'll see me again in three days. I felt like someone had kicked me in the stomach because I was totally convinced that I'd be seeing in the New Year, down the pub with my mates. When I came out of the meeting and walked back into the hall, Lucy looked up at me and could tell by the expression on my face, that the news wasn't good and as I made my way past her, she whispered, "Sorry John"

I went outside to the garden and walked up to one of the big round wooden park benches they had scattered around. I felt as if I wanted to scream and lifted the bench up with one hand and flipped it over, turning it upside down. I then went to the next one and did the same thing and the next, and the next.

"Don't lose it now John!" I kept telling myself, over and over again, "or I'll never get out of this fucking place and really will end up crazy!"

Looking up at the window at the top of the stairs, I could see Mo staring down at me.

"I've got to calm down!"

I took a deep breath and went back inside.

"Game of pool mate?" asked Zee as I entered the games room.

"Fuck it! Yeah, why not?"

I was trying to calm myself down but it wasn't working and told Zee that I wasn't in the mood to play any more. Leaving the games room, I walked slowly up to the other end of the hall and ripped a length of gold tinsel off the nurse's station window.

(Not much of a protest, I know)

Davina looked up from doing some paperwork and watched me as I turned around and walked down to the other end of the hall. Going up to the Christmas tree, I pulled one of the baubles off and crushed it under my foot and then turned around and walked up to the other end again, repeating the process several times. I felt like going mad and smashing the whole place to pieces but somehow managed to keep my rage bottled up inside, realising that would have made things much worse.

SECTION 2: MEDIUM

Davina came out of the nurse's station and said, "John, I brought those decorations in for the patients. Stop what you're doing right now!"

That made me feel a bit bad but I wasn't able to find it inside of me to apologise and so I went outside for another smoke and tried to calm myself down.

After dinner and Amanda, the night duty nurse was administering the meds. We were all lined up as usual and after I'd given mine to John in the games room, I walked back into the hall and watched the rest of the patients take theirs. For some strange reason, Lucy was still sitting down at a dining table (she always took her medication) and when the last of the patients had been given their prescribed drugs, Amanda called out to Lucy to come and take hers.

"No," she replied, "I don't want them!"

"Lucy, I told you to come and take your medication!" said Amanda in a stern voice.

There was something about Amanda that I couldn't take to; she seemed to be a really arrogant person and I could feel my blood starting to boil inside.

"Leave her alone," I called out, "she doesn't want them!"

Amanda ignored me and said, "Lucy, get over hear now!"

"LEAVE HER ALONE!" I yelled.

Lucy got up and stormed off into the lady's wing, with her arms crossed tightly across her chest.

"Lucy!" yelled Amanda, "Get back hear now!"

In a rage, I walked over to Amanda and screamed, "I SAID LEAVE HER ALONE, SHE DOESN'T WANT HER FUCKING MEDICATION!"

I could tell she was beginning to panic and Davina was helping Maria to have a bath, so she was on her own.

"John, keep out of this!" she yelled at me, clearly losing her temper.

"DON'T TREAT HER LIKE A LITTLE KID, SHE'S A GROWN WOMAN!"

"You're the one who's behaving like a child, don't be so immature!" she replied.

"FUCK YOU!" I screamed and stormed off back to my bedroom (Just like a little kid!)

Derek was fast asleep and snoring loudly, which for once was a comforting sound (at least he was still breathing!)

I was shaking with rage and had to go over to the window and have a cigarette, to calm myself down. My mobile phone rang and it was my cousin Mick on the other end.

"Hey John, how you doing mate, any news on your release date?"

I burst out crying and could tell it was really upsetting him.

"Oh John," was all he could say.

I managed to gather my composure and explained to him about the review going bad on me. He told me to try and keep my spirits up and would visit with Lee in a couple of day's time. I stayed in my room for the next three hours, talking to John who'd come in to see if I was alright. Derek woke up at one point and he seemed a little bit better and said that he was definitely going to have the operation.

When I asked him what had changed his mind, he said that he had to be brave for his family and realised that he'd been selfish. I couldn't wait to see Melanie and

SECTION 2: MEDIUM

tell her the news. Walking over to Derek's stereo, I put one of his Jerry Lee Lewis C.D's on for him and smoked about six fags, one after the other. When I eventually came out of our room, the hall was deserted apart from Zee sitting at a dining table, drinking a cup of coffee. Davina had finished her shift and Victor was in the nurse's station, talking to Amanda. They both stared at me as I walked across the hall and sat down next to Zee. Victor walked out of the nurse's station, sat down in a chair about twenty feet away from us, with a clipboard in his hand and wrote some things down from time to time while looking up at me all the while.

CHAPTER 34

New Years Day 2009, 12:00am and ten seconds.

Dominique was still up watching the celebrations at Trafalgar Square, on the television. She seemed very subdued, as were me and Zee. He was trying to conceal it but we could see Victor sending someone a text on his mobile phone (probably a family member, wishing them a "Happy New Year")
Amanda was in the nurse's station, on the telephone and laughing about something. Zee turned to me and said, "Happy New Year son," in the least cheerful tone you could imagine.
"Yeah, and you boy," I replied in an equally unenthusiastic manner.
Dominique switched off the T.V and walked past us saying, "Fuck this place, I'm going back to bed!"
It was just us two again and even though there was fuck all to do; we stayed up and talked about all the 'normal' people out there right now, getting pissed.

It was about one in the morning and Zee was fast asleep, with his arms folded under his head, hunched over the table. Amanda and Victor were doing the rounds of the lady's and men's wings, checking everyone was asleep and Zee was snoring quietly. Just then, the main door buzzed and Lucy walked into the hall holding her arm and made her way towards the games room. Just before she went inside, she turned

SECTION 2: MEDIUM

around and said in a quiet voice, "Can you come here a minute John?"

She then walked into the games room without turning the light on and I followed her, switching the light on as I went.

"What's wrong Luce, where have you been?" I asked.

She put her arm out and I could see a shard of glass sticking out of her wrist and blood pouring down to her elbow.

"For fuck's sake, what's happened?!"

"A man attacked me," she whispered.

"Zee! Zee! For fuck's sake, get in here now!" I screamed.

"What man? Where?"

Lucy looked up at me with tears in her eyes and said, "I had to get out of here for a while and this man came up to me....he was drunk"

Zee stood at the games room doorway, still half asleep.

"What's the matter?" he asked and then saw the pool of blood on the floor. "Fucking hell!"

"Go and get Victor, now!" I yelled and Zee ran off in the direction of the men's wing, shouting, "Victor, Victor, get here now!"

I sat Lucy down in a chair and lifted her arm up to try and stem the flow of blood.

"Come on, fucking hurry up!" yelled Zee and Victor strolled slowly up to me and Lucy and took a look at her arm. Amanda appeared in the doorway and Victor turned to her and told her to get some people up from Sherrin.

"What the fuck are you talking about!" screamed Zee, "She needs to see a fucking doctor!"

"Calm down and go to bed," said Victor.

"GET HER A FUCKING DOCTOR!" said Zee and started kicking the games room door in temper.

I was getting really angry at Victor because he didn't seem to have any sense of urgency about him.

"Fucking wake up you dozy cunt and get a doctor in here now!" I shouted at him.

He looked at me and then towards Amanda, who ran off to the nurse's station.

"CUNTS! YOU'RE ALL A LOAD OF FUCKING USELESS CUNTS!" screamed Zee and started punching the walls. It was the first time I'd ever seen Victor looking nervous and he didn't know which of us to speak to first.

"John, we are dealing with it, calm down"

"GET A FUCKING DOCTOR, THERE'S BLOOD EVERYWHERE!"

"Calm down John!"

"FUCKING CALM DOWN?" screamed Zee, "YOU NEED TO LIVEN UP, YOU CUNT!"

At that moment, two orderlies from Sherrin came rushing into the games room and grabbed hold of me and Zee. One of them pushed Zee up against the wall and the other held me down in the chair next to Lucy's, pinning my arms to the rests. Amanda came over with a towel and wrapped it around Lucy's wrist, being careful not to dislodge the glass and then led her out of the games room, into the hall. All of a sudden, Zee managed to break free and ran after Amanda, screaming, "WHERE ARE YOU FUCKING TAKING HER?"

The orderly pinning me down, let go and rushed out into the hall with his colleague. They both made a grab for Zee and crashed into one of the dining tables, scattering chairs all over the place. I got up and ran

SECTION 2: MEDIUM

into the hall, shouting at them to leave Zee alone and to get a doctor for Lucy. Victor pressed his panic button and stopped me from trying to help Zee. He grabbed hold of me and pushed me down onto one of the dining table chairs.

"Stay there!" he said, keeping his hands pressed down on my shoulders.

Zee managed to wriggle free again and ran after Amanda, who was opening the main entrance door with her other arm around Lucy. She just managed to get out of the way in time, when two more orderlies came rushing through the door and knocked Zee to the ground. One of them pinned his arms behind his back and the other pushed his knee down on the back of Zee's neck.

"Keep fucking still!" he yelled and this time, Zee wasn't going anywhere.

The other two orderlies got up and went with Amanda and Lucy and I could see them heading for the stairs, in the direction of Sherrin.

"WHERE ARE YOU FUCKING GOING!" I yelled, "SHE NEEDS TO SEE A FEMALE DOCTOR! SHE DOESN'T LIKE MEN TOUCHING HER!"

The orderly who had his knee on Zee's neck, got to his feet and walked over to me.

"Shut your mouth you little prick, or you'll end up in there with her!" he said.

The other orderly pulled Zee up from the floor and slammed him into a chair next to me.

"Don't fucking move!"

A nurse walked in and handed me a tablet and a glass of water and then looked at the orderly who said, "Swallow that pill, before I ram it down your fucking throat!"

I did as I was told and then the orderly pulled my mouth open and yelled at me to run my tongue around my gums, between my teeth. When he was satisfied that I'd swallowed the tablet, he did exactly the same thing to Zee.

Vincent and these two orderlies then went into the nurse's station and sat there, watching us through the glass. I couldn't stand the fact that they'd drugged me up and had coffee after coffee, for the rest of the night and eventually ended up going to bed at about seven in the morning.

I woke up at three in the afternoon and went out into the hall. There was no sign of Zee and so I walked into the games room, expecting to find him there but once again, there was no sign of him. I looked down at the floor to see if the blood was still there but it was spotless and for a second, I thought I'd dreamt the whole thing until I noticed a small blood stain on the chair where Lucy had been sitting. I walked straight into the nurse's station, where Mo, Nelson and the young female nurse were on duty and asked, "What's happened to Lucy?"

All three of them ignored me and carried on doing their paperwork, so I went to the drawer and got my cigarettes and lighter out for myself and went downstairs for a smoke. After about the third cigarette, I walked into the downstairs lobby and saw Stewart coming out of the doors which led to Sherrin. He saw me but tried to carry on walking past.

"Stewart, Stewart!" I said, "How's Lucy? How's her arm?"

"She's okay; they said she did it just for attention"

SECTION 2: MEDIUM

"But she had a lump of glass sticking out of her wrist!"
"It looked worse than it was, she never hit any veins"
He looked so calm but I couldn't understand why and he was beginning to annoy me.
"She said she was attacked last night. Has a doctor examined her?" I asked.
He just stared at me, saying nothing and smiled politely.
"Stewart"
"What?"
"Was she raped last night?"
Silence.
"Stewart!"
"What John?"
"Was she raped?"
"Yes" he replied calmly.
I felt sick in the stomach.
"Where's your fucking God now!" I said and stormed off.

CHAPTER 35

After dinner I sat down at a table with Maz and Zee. I thought they had sent him back to Sherrin but it turned out he was so drugged up, he'd slept to about five in the afternoon. I told him and Maz, what Stewart had told me and they couldn't believe it. My mobile phone started to ring and it was the salesman from the Smart garage, asking how I was getting on with the car and was I pleased with it. I told him where I was and he started laughing, thinking I was joking. When I told him that I was being serious, he was shocked and said that when I got discharged, to go and see him. After meds, my father-in-law came to visit me. He's one of the nicest blokes you could ever meet and we had always got on really well. He brought me in some books to read and a bar of chocolate. A packet of fags would have been nicer! (Only joking mate)

We went into the games room where it was quiet and sat down. I could tell he was feeling awkward and it must have been really hard for him, what with me splitting up with his daughter. I told him that she was making it purposely difficult for me to see my daughter and showed him a letter from her solicitor, stating that I had to see her under supervision in a rough area of London. It would have been a ten mile drive away when I could have seen her in the next town from my village and in much nicer surroundings.

"There's no way I want my daughter to be in the same room with a load of drug addicts and low life's," I thought (I must sound like a right snob)

SECTION 2: MEDIUM

My father-in-law tried to convince me that my wife would never do that but I was having none of it and yet we still managed to say goodbye on good terms. He could obviously tell I didn't have a fucking clue what I was talking about and was totally confused. I found out later that the solicitor had made a mistake and put in the wrong address of the place where I was supposed to see my daughter but I still felt angry towards my wife.

"Why did I have to see my little girl under supervision?" I thought.

It felt like I was some sort of evil person who wanted to do harm to her and that's the last thing in the world I would ever do. In fact, if I ever saw someone trying to hurt or abduct any kid, I'd kill them in the blink of an eye.

That evening and the only people up were Zee, Maz, Dominique and myself. There had been no sign of Lucy all day and we hadn't heard any more news either. Zee and Maz were playing pool in the games room, while Dominique was sitting on her own at one of the dining tables in the hall, drinking a cup of coffee. I went to the vending machine and got a coffee for myself and then sat down next to her. She was very quiet and I think the news of Lucy had really affected her.

"I was thinking about walking out of this place last night," she said, "I'm glad I didn't"

"She was in the wrong place at the wrong time"

"Who did it?" she asked.

"I dunno, it must have been some drunken reveller walking home from somewhere. There would have been a lot of them about last night"

"Fucking bastard!"

2nd January, 8am.

I noticed Stewart coming out of Sherrin while I was having a cigarette and when he saw me, he came outside to join me.
"How is she?" I asked.
"She's very quiet but seems to be comfortable"
"Why have they got her in there, she's done nothing wrong?"
"It's for her own safety. They're afraid she might try to harm herself again and can keep her under closer supervision in Sherrin"
"Those fucking orderlies were useless! Me and Zee were screaming at them to get Lucy to a doctor and they didn't seem to care!"
"Victor took one look at the glass sticking out of her wrist and knew she'd been careful where to put it" he said.
"What?"
"She's done it loads of times. She doesn't want to kill herself and yet she sometimes wishes she were dead"
"I don't understand"
"It's a cry for help but help never comes…..well, not until she found God"
I started to see why Lucy had so much faith in God. All her adult life, none of the doctors had been able to help her but she found some kind of peace in religion and that's why Stewart was the ideal man for her.
"She's still a virgin you know" he whispered.
"But she can't be, she…….."
"She never gave consent and I doubt if she ever will"
"They should have still taken her to see a doctor….after what that bastard did"

SECTION 2: MEDIUM

Maz was due to have his review at eleven. His mum and dad went in with him and after about half an hour, he came out with Tina who sat down next to him on the sofa by the main exit. I walked up to them and smiled at Tina before asking Maz how it went.
"They don't think I'm ready yet," he replied, "and feel I might be suicidal"
"Are you?"
"I don't know"
Tina wrote something down on the clipboard she was carrying and then went into the nurse's station and started talking to Davina.
"Where's your mum and dad now?" I asked.
"The doctor wanted a word with them in private and told me to wait out here"
He was looking depressed and I was worried about him.
"Don't do anything stupid," I said.
Zee called me into the games room for a game of pool and Dominique was playing on the Xbox with Craig. She seemed a lot happier today and turned her gaze away from the T.V to look at me.
"Hey John, are you finally gonna get to fucking draw me today?" she asked.
"Oh shit yeh, sorry mate… I forgot all about it. I'll do it tonight and that's a definite"
She turned back to the T.V screen.
"Good" she said.
Me and Zee were half way through a game when we heard shouting coming from the hall.
"What the fuck's going on out there?" said Zee and put his pool cue on the table and went out to have a look. I followed him into the hall and Craig and Dominique went over to the window that overlooked

the doctor's car park. She was laughing like crazy while Craig started shouting, "CUNT, CUNT, CUNT!" over and over again.
It was the first time I'd seen him excited about something, let alone swear.
"What is it?" I called out.
"Quick, come back in here and look out the window!" yelled Dominique.
I ran back into the games room with Zee.
"Go on Maz, run!" she yelled. "Don't let them fuckers catch you!"
I looked out of the window and saw Maz running down the street, followed by Davina and three orderlies from Sherrin. It looked like something from The Benny Hill Show and we all burst out laughing and shouted, "Go Maz, go!"
Maz's mum and dad came rushing out of the review room with the doctor and even Maz's dad seemed to be trying to conceal a smile. It was obviously something Maz had done before and in no time at all, he was back in the ward and treated like a king by Zee, for the rest of the day.

After giving my lunch time meds to John, I took a stroll along the men's corridor to pay Tina a visit (she was doing the suicide watch outside Ennio's room again)
I walked up to her, leant forward and kissed her firmly on the lips as she put her hand round the back of my neck and held me there for a few seconds. I then handed her a slip of paper with my phone number on it, squeezed her hand and walked back to the main hall. After Nigel was discharged, Chris moved into his room and I suppose they felt with him shitting himself

all night, he wouldn't disturb anyone else if he were in a single room. No sooner had he moved, his old bed was taken over by a new guy (after they had changed the sheets!) who must have been in his late forties. I remember him walking into the hall for the first time and he looked completely shocked, like a rabbit caught in the headlights of a car.

Mental illness was something that I hadn't really taken that seriously but since I'd been admitted into the hospital, my outlook had changed completely. It could affect anyone and this place was full of patients with some kind or other (accept for Chris and his brain damage) and looking back on my time in there, I realise that I've become so much more aware of all the different mental and physical illnesses that some people suffer from.

After lunch, a man and woman arrived in smart suits and they followed Victoria and Mo into the men's wing. I looked over at Tina who was in the nurse's station and mouthed silently, "Who are they?"

She came out of the doorway, walked over to me and whispered, "They're from the Italian consulate. They've arranged for Ennio to be flown home and have come to take him to the airport"

"So he's been discharged?"

"Not exactly. More that he's been signed over and transferred to a hospital in Italy"

"What about his mum and dad, where are they?"

"I think they're going to meet him at the airport when he lands back in Italy" she replied.

Tina then went back to the nurse's station and sat down at the desk, to do some paperwork. Dominique and Zee were sitting with me and as we were talking amongst ourselves, Ennio appeared from the men's corridor with Mo and Victoria either side of him and the two Italians following behind.

As they walked past our table, he stopped and gave me back my iPod and whispered, "Thank you John," in clear English.

I gave him a hug, smiled and wished him good luck.

Zee shook his hand and said in a deep voice, "See you later son"

Dominique kissed him on the cheek and gave him a great big squeeze. They all then walked into the nurse's station to fill out some paperwork and then he was gone….as quick as that. I looked over at Dominique and notice that she had tears in her eyes and I started to laugh quietly to myself.

"What's so funny?" she asked, wiping the tears away with the back of her hand.

"Nothing mate," I replied, "nothing at all"

My sister Pauline and Dave came to visit me that evening and we went into the games room to talk. They both took turns in the massage chair and I reckon Pauline could have stayed there all night long. I played a couple of games of pool with Dave and was surprised how calm and relaxed he appeared to be. Most of the visitors I'd observed, seemed to be on edge and uncomfortable but being in this place didn't appear to faze him at all. (I did finally get to understand why, seven months later)

Zee, Dominique and Maz were in the games room with us and when I wanted to go for a cigarette, I felt totally at ease leaving them with my sister and brother-in-law. There wasn't anybody else outside in

the courtyard and as I smoked my cigarette, I looked over to the caged area of Sherrin and wondered how Lucy was getting on. After Pauline and Dave had left, Maz and Dominique were looking at the picture I'd put up on the wall of our art gallery and Maz was raving about it, asking lots of questions about what all of the images meant.
"Do you really like it?" I asked him.
"Yeh, its fucking brilliant!"
I went and got a pen and wrote on it, "To Maz, from your friend John"
"It's yours now," I told him.
"Fucking hell John, are you sure?"
"One hundred percent"
Since the incident with Lucy, something had happened to me. The feeling that I was somehow smarter and superior to everyone else was starting to become less and less prominent and I no longer felt that my picture was that good or I was that good at art either.
"Are you going to draw me now?" asked Dominique.
I really wasn't in the mood but had promised her I would.
"Come on then," I replied.
While I went to get a sketch pad and a pencil, she went over to the sofa by the nurse's station and sprawled herself out across it. I really didn't feel like drawing her but gave it a go anyway and as she posed and pouted, Victor walked by every now and then and told me it was good. When I'd finished, I gave it to Dominique and she seemed pleased with it and said she was going to stick it on the wall above her bed.

Two in the morning and I was in the games room with the lights off, having a cigarette by the slightly open window. After eleven at night, smoking was not allowed outside and it definitely wasn't permitted inside either. I would always have the hand holding the cigarette, squeezed through the open gap so that the smoke wouldn't fill the room and lent on the window ledge casually, as if I were just gazing at the view outside. By staring into the window pane, I could see the hall behind me reflected in the glass and saw the timid nurse I'd told to get out of the men's wing, walking towards the games room door. As she entered the room, I flicked the cigarette as far as I could and carried on staring out the window, as if I hadn't noticed her.

"John, smoking is not allowed in the building," she said.

Without turning around, I answered, "I'm not smoking"

"I can smell it from out in the hall"

"I'm not smoking," I repeated and turned around and walked past her to get a coffee from the vending machine. She said something about not smoking again and went back to the nurse's station. Dominique was the only other patient still up and she was sitting at the dining table nearest to the Christmas tree. After getting myself a coffee, I went over and sat down next to her.

"Can't sleep?" I said.

"Nah….. but Victor can," she replied.

"What do you mean?"

"He's locked himself in the quiet room and is fast asleep on the sofa. Come and have a look"

The light was switched off in the quiet room but looking through the window, I could just about make out Victor stretched out on the sofa with a blanket draped over him. Dominique slammed the palm of her hand on the door several times and yelled out, "Wakey, wakey. Time to get up, you lazy fucker!"

I started to laugh and banged the side of my fist on the door a couple of times but didn't say anything. I couldn't swear at Victor, I respected him too much for that but his relaxed attitude the other night when Zee was yelling out for him to come and see Lucy annoyed me. It's only now as I'm writing this and thinking back, that I realise why he had been so calm that night. As Stewart had said, Lucy made a habit of either cutting or sticking sharp objects in her wrists. When Victor had seen it wasn't serious, he kept his cool in order to try and calm down me and Zee. If he'd started to panic, then it would have made matters much worse.

"Fucking wake up, you cunt!" shouted Dominique and she started laughing loudly.

I couldn't stop laughing either and banged my fist on the door again.

"Who is that? Stop it!" came a deep, gruff voice from inside the quiet room.

The timid nurse came out of the nurse's station and told me and Dominique to get to bed.

"Not until Victor gets up," said Dominique, "he's supposed to be on night duty, watching us lot!" and with that, she gave another loud bang on the quiet room door.

"Stop it!" called out Victor and then he opened the door and walked back to the nurse's station. Dominique was about to follow him and give some more abuse but I grabbed her by the arm and told her that she'd done enough. He was awake now and doing what he was supposed to be doing, she'd won. I went back to bed and briefly thought about my review the next day but didn't hold out much hope after the incident with Lucy on New Year's morning. I had become resigned to the fact that I'd be here for some time to come and the best thing I could do was not to cause any trouble.

3rd January, 7am.

I was queuing up to get my breakfast and saw Maria walk out from the lady's wing, followed by Sarah who still had the bandage wrapped around her head.
Sarah fell over again but this time, landed on her hands and knees and didn't seem to have hurt herself. Victor strolled over to her and calmly told her to get up. She didn't respond and so he grabbed a chair from one of the dining tables and put it in front of her and told her to grab hold of it and pull herself up. She slowly stretched out her arm and grabbed hold of one of the chair legs and was clearly struggling to move, while Victor stood next to the chair and towered above her. To me, it was a sickening sight. There was this great big able-bodied bloke standing there and he wasn't allowed to hold on to her or lift her up because of health and safety regulations. Not only might he hurt her if she was injured in some way but he also might have strained his back in the process of helping her up. Victor was like a fucking giant and could have picked her up with one arm but wasn't allowed to. I felt like going over there myself and helping Sarah up but decided it was best not to. I didn't want to do anything that might mess up my review at eleven and so like everyone else in the hall, I watched Sarah struggle slowly to her feet and sit down on the chair.

SECTION 2: MEDIUM

Victor saw me looking over at him and I could see he felt ashamed that he wasn't allowed to help her but rules were rules. There was still no sign of Lucy back on the ward and so I went downstairs for a cigarette, in the hope of seeing Stewart coming out of the doors leading to Sherrin.

Melanie was outside smoking in the blind spot and she seemed to be in a good mood. I told her what Derek had said to me about him agreeing to have the operation and she said that she already knew and it was scheduled for a couple of days time. She asked me if I was ready for my review and after replying that I was, she explained that she'd meet me back here at a quarter to eleven and then went back upstairs to see some of the other patients. Stewart walked out of the Sherrin doors with Lucy and they were carrying a load of bags. I walked up to them and asked, "Are you going back upstairs to our ward?"

Lucy smiled at me and answered, "No....I've been discharged; I'm going home with Stewart"

I look at Stewart who nodded.

"It's true," he said with a smile on his face.

I couldn't believe it, I thought she'd be in there for a long time to come but I guess the doctors felt she would be much better off living with Stewart. We exchanged phone numbers and after shaking Stewart's hand and giving Lucy a hug goodbye, they were gone.

I never saw Lucy again.

Zee and Maz were playing pool in the games room when I got back upstairs and I joined them for a couple of games.

"You've got your review at eleven, ain't you?" asked Zee.

"Yeah," I replied, not feeling at all confident about the outcome.

"Looks like I won't be getting out of here any time soon," said Maz.

"Not after you done a runner!" laughed Zee and took his shot. I told them both that Lucy had been discharged and they were both surprised, Zee even more so. Melanie stuck her head round the games room doorway at twenty to eleven and asked if I wanted to go down for a cigarette.

"Does the pope wear a funny hat?!"

When we were outside, she told me that she'd do most of the talking in the review and I didn't argue. I couldn't think of anything to say to the doctors that I thought would help towards my discharge and wasn't feeling in the least bit hopeful. We went into the review at exactly eleven o'clock and Nelson was there with two doctors. I spent most of the time staring out the window, while Melanie talked on my behalf and I answered yes and no at the appropriate places. Finally, the doctor addressed me and said, "Well John, I think you are ready to be discharged"

I thought I'd misheard him and looked over to Melanie who was smiling. I hadn't been listening to what she had said to them but what ever it was, it worked.

"When can I leave?" was all I could say.

"We want you to spend one more night with us and then you can leave tomorrow at noon. That will give you time to arrange transport back home and to get all your things together," replied the doctor.

When we walked back outside to the hall, I thanked Melanie for all she had done for me and she gave me a hug and wished me all the best. Dominique was sitting on the sofa by the nurse's station and when I told her that I was leaving tomorrow, she replied, "You lucky fuck!" and kissed me on the cheek.

After meds that evening, Mo asked me if I would mind spending my last night upstairs in the other ward as they were expecting a new patient that night and felt he'd be better suited to our ward. I agreed and went back to my bedroom to grab my stash of cigarettes and my toothbrush and toothpaste. It's funny but although I had spent only three weeks in hospital, so much had happened in that ward and it felt as if I was leaving home for the evening. The ward upstairs was laid out completely different to ours and was only half full. Mo had told me that it was mainly used by patients who were either deemed to be low risk or were due to be discharged in the near future. My new bedroom consisted of six beds and apart from mine, only one other was occupied. This bed had the curtains drawn around it and someone was sleeping soundly inside. I put my toothbrush and toothpaste on the cabinet next to my bed and went for a look around the ward, to see if there was anywhere I could have a crafty cigarette. I thought it was best not to smoke outside the bedroom window, as I didn't know the routine here and didn't know if a member of staff made regular visits to the bedrooms, to check on the patients. I was due to be discharged the next day and the last thing I needed was to mess it all up by getting caught smoking. I walked down the corridor and came to a room on my left, which had two arcade machines in it. After plugging them in, I started playing on this old fashioned driving game and kept an eye on the window, to see if an orderly walked past. I'd kept the light switched off so I could only be seen by the glow from the arcade machine and out of the corner of my eye; I spotted someone peering through the window at me. I pretended not to have seen them and after a short while, they walked away and carried on down the hall and so I immediately went over to the window and sparked up a cigarette. From the slightly open window, I could see my other ward downstairs going off at a right angle to this part of the building. All the lights were off and I imagined Zee and the rest of the guys, tucked up and fast asleep in their beds. I was starting to feel tired myself and so after finishing the cigarette and flicking it out of the window; I went back to my room, drew the curtains round the bed and fell fast asleep.

In the morning after brushing my teeth, I asked the orderly on duty if I could go back to my ward. He rang downstairs and said that I could and so I made my own way back, having a cigarette at the smoking area on the way. Tina was on duty and she waved to me as I walked past the nurse's station to get a coffee from the vending machine. I then sat at one of the dining tables, waiting for everyone to get up. Part of me felt as if I'd beaten the system because in all the time I was in the hospital, I'd never taken any medication apart from the night when the orderly from Sherrin practically rammed it down my throat. It's strange but you'd think I could remember vividly, finally being discharged but I can't recall any of it. I can't remember who came to pick me up or saying goodbye to any of the guys and the only thing I do remember is giving Maria a hug, just before walking out the main door for the last time.

SECTION 3: LOW

CHAPTER 36

Someone had obviously dropped me back at my flat and I can't believe they would have left me on my own straight away but now it was early evening and I sat at the table in my kitchen, surrounded by burning candles and not knowing what I was going to do next. The electric meter was nearly empty and I didn't have a penny to my name. There was a knock at the door and when I opened it, I was surprised to see my friend Darren the window cleaner.
"Hiya Darren. Wanna come in?"
He just stood there with a worried expression on his face.
"Where have you been John? I haven't seen you for ages. I got the Christmas present you gave me!"
Before being sectioned, I was walking along the high street one day and stopped to talk to Darren, who was cleaning the window of the chemists. He pointed to a digital camera behind the glass and said that he was going to try and save up for it. It was only £20 (some foreign name I'd never heard of) and it could record up to thirty minutes of video.
"I can use it to make my own films, just like you said you wanted to do," he explained.
I spoke to him for a bit longer and then said I had to go. One of my neighbours worked in the chemist and I knocked on her door that night and gave her the £20, asking if she'd save it for me. She said that Darren had already asked if she could not sell it to anyone else

and I explained it was going to be a Christmas present for him.

"I'll take it out the window," she replied, "and when he asks where it is, I'll say that someone else sold it on the day I wasn't working"

Now as Darren stood on my doorstep, I realised that my neighbour must have given him the camera while I was in hospital. I'd forgotten all about it.

"Come in mate, it's fucking freezing out there! You're letting all the cold air in" I said.

Darren took off his donkey jacket and sat on the sofa.

"Where were you John? I missed you"

"I spent the Christmas break with my family in Hampshire," I lied.

He nodded and I think he believed me and then got the camera out of his jacket pocket.

"Do you like it?" I asked.

"You have to have a computer to watch anything on it and I haven't got one. Can you plug it into yours and show me how it works?"

"Oh for fuck's sake!" I thought, "I wish I'd never bought him the fucking thing!"

Just at that moment, there was a knock on the door. It was the crisis team; a man and a woman I recognised but didn't know their names. They had told me in the hospital that they'd be around that evening but I'd forgotten.

"Hello John, can we come in?" asked the man.

"Yeh, of course. Budge up Darren"

"Oh, you've got company," said the man. "Is this an okay time?"

"Yeh, yeh, no worries. Sit yourselves down"

I looked at Darren and could see he was worried. He must have had dealings with these sorts of people

before. He got up from the sofa and grabbed his coat.
"I'm gonna be going now John," he said.
"No, no, don't be silly," I replied.
"Perhaps it would be better if we do speak in private," said the woman.
"No, he's alright, ain't you Darren? Sit down on one of the dining table chairs"
"I'd better be going"
"Sit down!"
Darren did as I said and the two crisis team members sat on the sofa.
"Well John," asked the man, "How are you feeling?"
"I'm feeling just great, aren't I Darren?"
With that, Darren shot out of his chair and ran out of the flat without as much as a bye or leave.
"Cheers mate," I murmured to myself, "Thanks for the support"
The rest of the meeting was filled with a load of mundane crap I can't recall but all I can remember saying was that I was skint. The crisis team had given me a number to ring if I needed any assistance and said they would pay me daily visits for the next two weeks. After spending three weeks amongst all that noise and mayhem, my flat felt deathly quiet and I couldn't stand being on my own. A crisis loan was available to any patients who didn't have any money but I didn't feel like ringing them and rather wanted to see them in person and so after the man and woman left, I got in my car and drove back to the hospital.

It was 8pm and when I walked into the reception area of the mental health part of the hospital, there was no one about and so I went over to the door that led to our ward and pressed the intercom. While I was waiting

for a reply, I looked above my head and saw a camera pointing down at me. The staff in my ward knew I was back and I wondered what their reaction would be. Victor's voice came over the intercom, "What do you want John?"
"I want to see a member of the crisis team. I haven't got any money and need a loan"
"There is no one here, they have all gone home," he replied.
"What's the fucking point of having a crisis loan for patients, when there ain't anyone around to give it to you?"
"Come back in the morning and a member of the team will see you"
"I haven't got enough petrol to go back home and then get back here tomorrow"
There was silence over the intercom.
"Hello Victor…….are you there, have you got any suggestions?"
"Go back home and the crisis team will contact you in the morning. They can arrange to come to your flat and see you," he finally replied.
"I haven't even got enough money for the gas meter and its fucking freezing!" I yelled and slammed my fist against the intercom speaker.
I walked around the reception area, swearing to myself and then remembered I had Maz's mobile phone number. He always had loads of money on him and so I gave him a ring.
"Maz, it's John," I said when he answered the call.
"Hey John, where are you?"
"I'm outside in the reception area. Could you lend me a fiver until I get some money from the crisis team? I

need it so I can put some money in the gas and electric meters"

"No problem, I'll be with you in a minute!" he said and then hung up.

A short while later, I heard the sound of running footsteps and shouting and so I went back over to the door leading to our ward. Maz appeared through the glass and he pressed the door release button and just managed to pass me a five pound note before Victor grabbed him round the waist.

"Cheers Maz," I said as he was dragged back down the corridor and the door clicked shut.

"Fuck all of you cunts!" he yelled and then I heard the buzzer sound to the entrance of our ward and after it shut; silence. I sent him a text, thanking him again and then drove back to the flat, stopping at a petrol station on the way back to get some change for the meters.

Back at the flat, my mobile beeped to say I had a message and when I opened it, I was surprised to see it was Tina. She said that she was on duty until eleven and would love to see me after work. I sent her back a text, giving the directions to my flat and then got a beer from the fridge (it had been there since before I was sectioned) and gulped it down in seconds. Unless you knew where I lived, it was pretty hard to find as it was down a small lane in between the two curry houses and was the first flat at the edge of a courtyard. Tina rang me as she was entering the village and I walked up to the main road and waved to her as she drew close by. When we got inside the flat, we embraced each other and must have held a kiss for about thirty seconds.

SECTION 3: LOW

"Won't your husband be wondering where you are?" I asked.
"He works nights and would have left the house before I got home" she replied.
"What about your ten year old son you mentioned, who's at home with him?"
"Charlene, my second daughter still lives at home and is keeping an eye on him"
"Won't she be wondering where you are?"
"I sent her a text to say that I'm staying at Davina's tonight"
The thought immediately went through my mind that she wanted to stay the night and then we kissed again and sat down on the sofa. I pulled her legs up onto the cushioned seat and lay on top of her and we kissed each other all over, for what seemed like ages. I eventually suggested that we go upstairs and we spent the next couple of hours in each others arms, pulling and grabbing at one another until I fell fast asleep, completely exhausted and without going all the way.

The next morning, Tina woke me with a cup of tea and was already dressed.
"I've got to go, I'm back on shift at nine," she said and kissed me on the lips.
"What time do you get off?"
"It's only a short shift. I finish at two but then I've got a hairdressers appointment at two thirty"
"I could meet you after your appointment and we could go for a coffee," I suggested.
"You told me last night that you said to Victor, you didn't have enough petrol to get back"

"I was just saying that as an excuse to try and get some money straight away. Is the hairdressers in the parade of shops near the hospital?"

"No," she replied, "it's at a friend's house; I've been using her for years. I'll ring you when she's nearly finished"

Tina then got a twenty pound note out of her purse and said, "Here, take this. You might need it just in case you haven't got enough petrol"

"I can't take that Tina"

"Take it," she said and pressed it into my hand before kissing me again and then going downstairs to her car. After she left, I got dressed and went over the road to the newsagents and with the twenty pounds, bought three packs of cigarettes. With the fiver change, I planned to get some petrol.

"My car's really economical and a fivers worth of fuel will last me ages," I convinced myself.

As I walked back to the flat, my mobile rang and it was someone asking if the crisis team could come and visit me in the next hour. I agreed and rushed back home. I'd become totally paranoid that they were not working on my behalf but were still trying to find out what was wrong with me.

"They're wasting their time," I said to myself, "I'm completely sane and if those fuckers think they can prove otherwise, then they've got another thing coming!"

Back in the flat, I pulled the T.V cabinet out of the way and dragged the sofa up against the wall before repositioning the T.V cabinet where the sofa had been. I then switched on the laptop and angled it so the camera above the screen, pointed directly at the sofa and then placed a piece of card over the screen. When they came and called at the door, all I had to do was press a button and I could film them interviewing me. It looked a bit strange with the T.V stuck in the middle of the room and so I pulled a load of DVD's off the shelf and scattered them all over the floor and if they asked, I'd tell them I was in the middle of rearranging the furniture.

My front doorbell rang while I was making a cup of black coffee (I wanted tea but didn't have enough money to buy some milk) and after pressing the record button, I answered it. The two members of the crisis team, who'd evaluated me with my brother when I'd asked to be admitted again, were standing there. I pointed to the sofa and asked them to take a seat and offered them both a black coffee, which they declined.

They asked me if I had been taking my medication since being discharged and I lied that I had.

"I need a crisis loan," I told them, "I haven't got any money"

Saviour, the black guy said in a strong African accent, "We are going to give you a crisis card and there are several phone numbers on the back, which you can ring. One of them is in regards to obtaining a temporary crisis loan"

The white lady looked around the living room and asked, "What's happening here then?"

"I'm having a change around and you've caught me in the middle of it"

They must have carried on asking me questions for about twenty minutes and the words went straight over my head. In my imagination, they were saying to themselves, "He's still sick, he needs to be taken back to the mental hospital, he's dangerous!"

"You're not gonna get anything over on me," I thought, "I'll have proof that you're trying to set me up!"

They both finally stood up and as I opened the door for them to leave, I pulled down the card covering the laptop screen and said, "Smile, you're on candid camera!"

The white lady seemed to find it amusing but Saviour definitely didn't.

"What is this all about," he said, "You have no right filming us!"

"This is my home and I can do whatever I want and now I want you both to leave!"

"This is very serious John and I don't take kindly to it at all. We will be back with a doctor this afternoon and with that, he marched out with the girl following close behind. After they'd gone, I wanted to make sure that I was within my rights to be able to film someone while they were in my home and so I looked it up on the internet and discovered that I was. I couldn't hang about the flat waiting for the crisis team to come back and so after tidying up the place (I took the Christmas tree out into the street, with all the decorations and lights still on it and threw it in the builder's skip) I then decided to drive back to the hospital and see them there. The five pounds worth of petrol took the tank to just over a quarter and I figured that if I drove carefully, it should last me a couple of days.

CHAPTER 37

When I got to the hospital, I found a parking place in the car park but didn't have any money for the machine and just hoped for the best.
There were two receptionists at the desk in the lobby and I asked one of them to call a member of the crisis team. She was hesitant at first but when I told her that I'd only been discharged the day before, she rang through to someone. My mobile phone beeped with a text message and it was Tina. It read:
'Somebody saw us kissing in the corridor the other night. I've got a disciplinary with Victoria. Don't know what to do!'
I couldn't believe what I was reading, who could have seen us? Was it Davina? No, it couldn't have been, she was supposed to be Tina's friend.
Maybe it was a patient, Dominique? John? Luke?
Shit, Tina was in real trouble and it was all my fault!
Melanie walked in the building and was surprised to see me.
"What are you doing back here, John?" she asked.
"I've come for a crisis loan, I'm skint!"
"You should have phoned them, they won't like it you being back here after being discharged…..and for the second time in three weeks!"
Saviour and his colleague came out of the door leading to the ward I'd been in and walked up to me and Melanie.

"We'd like to speak to you in our office John, please come with us" he said.

Melanie stepped in front of me and said, "I want to be present while you are questioning John"

"This doesn't concern you Melanie," he replied. "John has been discharged and is now in the hands of the crisis team"

"While he is still under the care of the NHS, I am still his advocate. If you don't allow me in that room with him, then he's not going in"

I felt so proud of her and was amazed at how much authority she had.

Saviour turned to his female colleague and she just shrugged her shoulders and gave a slight nod.

When we got into the office, the doctor who'd assessed me during my reviews was sitting down on a sofa and he had a serious expression on his face. Me and Melanie sat down opposite him and you could tell that he wasn't happy at her being there.

"Why have you come back here John?"

"I need a crisis loan, I haven't got any money!"

"The crisis team here," he said, gesturing in the direction of Saviour and his colleague, "explained the proper procedures to you, regarding how to go about obtaining a crisis loan"

"Yeh, I know but……"

"And they told me that you filmed them while they were speaking to you, without their permission"

Melanie looked at me and then back at the doctor, totally confused.

"It is an illegal offence to make recordings of individuals without their consent and I want you to give me the tape please"

"I did it on my laptop, there isn't any tape and it's not illegal if you are in your own home," I replied.
"How do you know this?"
"I looked it up on the government's website and it states that you are perfectly entitled to use any recording equipment in your own home, unless it breaches any copyright laws"
"I don't take kindly to having conversations of a professional manner, being secretly recorded and want you to erase it"
"I already have"
"I beg your pardon?"
"I already have. After they left, I listened back to it and there wasn't anything I thought would be useful to me"
"What do you mean, useful?"
"I thought they were trying to get me sectioned again"
He stayed quiet for a moment and wrote something down on a clipboard on his lap. Finally, he said, "I want another doctor to see you. She is totally impartial and does not work for this hospital but is here today, speaking to other members of our team. How do you feel about that?"
"I don't mind," I replied.
"Good. Please wait outside in the reception area and we'll call you when she is ready to see you"
"Where is he going to be evaluated?" asked Melanie.
The doctor looked at the crisis team, then at me and then at Melanie.
"In Sherrin Ward," he said bluntly.

"What the fuck is wrong with you John, are you mad?" whispered Melanie as we sat outside in the lobby.

"Of course I'm mad, that's why they sectioned me"

"Don't play games with these people John….it's not a joking matter"

"What's the big deal?" I replied, "I've already been discharged, they can't do anything to me"

She shook her head and explained, "You're still under the care of the mental health team and if they feel that you need to be sectioned again, they will do it!"

"But I haven't done anything wrong; I've only come to get a crisis loan"

"You've really pissed them off by recording those two members of the crisis team. What were you playing at, what were you trying to prove?"

I shrugged my shoulders and didn't reply, I had no answer. Just at that moment, Victoria came through the door, followed by Tina and both of them didn't look happy. As they walked past, Victoria spotted me and gave me a filthy look. Tina looked really upset and looked at me with tears in her eyes.

"Keep walking!" said Victoria in a stern voice and they both went through another door on the opposite side of the lobby.

"What was that all about?" asked Melanie.

"I think she's in a lot of trouble"

"Why, what's happened?"

"Somebody saw me and Tina kissing the other night and has reported it"

"You have got to be kidding me, right?"

"I'm afraid not," I answered in a quiet voice.

"And this happened on the ward, while she was on duty?"

"Yes"

"Why didn't you tell me all this before?"

"I didn't think I needed to"

SECTION 3: LOW

"This isn't good John, they can use all of this against you and what worries me the most is the doctor wants to assess you in Sherrin"

Saviour and the other member of the crisis team appeared and asked me and Melanie to follow them. We went outside and walked to the bottom of the staff car park and then turned left at the end of the building. A narrow road sloped slightly downwards to another, smaller car park and running alongside it was Sherrin Ward. We walked up to a steel black door and Saviour pressed a button on the intercom. From the inside, I could hear two sets of doors being unlocked before a buzzing noise sounded and then someone over the intercom told us we could go in. There was an orderly I recognised from the caged smoking area, standing inside the doorway and as we walked past him, he nodded to me. We immediately went through another door, which the orderly locked behind us and through a final door (locked again)

I was standing in a brightly lit, square shaped room and there was a reception desk to one side with a female member of staff behind it. A middle-aged lady in a smart suit was leaning on the counter of the desk, writing something down and Melanie gave me a gentle nudge with her elbow.

"I fucking know her," she whispered, "she was the doctor in charge of me at Cranbridge and she's a right bitch!"

The orderly unlocked a door to our left and told me and Melanie to go through and then locked us inside. We were in this small room with a round table and four blue chairs surrounding it, in the middle of the floor. At the end of the room there was a single bed with a black rubber mattress but without any sheets or pillows. I sat down on one of the chairs and tried to pull it forward, nearer to the table but it wouldn't budge. Looking down at the base, I noticed that it was bolted to the floor as were all the other chairs as well as the table.

Melanie saw me looking around the room and said, "Anything than can be picked up and thrown, is bolted down in this place"

I looked at the windows and they were covered with metal bars and the glass had wire mesh inside, to stop anyone smashing it and using the glass as a weapon. Suddenly, the door unlocked and the lady doctor walked in with the two crisis team members and the orderly. There weren't enough seats for us all, so Saviour went over to the bed and sat down, while his female colleague sat opposite me and Melanie, next to the doctor and finally, the orderly stood in front of the door with his arms crossed. The doctor recognised Melanie immediately and nodded to her but didn't say anything and then turned her attention to me.

"Hello John, I'm Doctor Jefferson. Before I start, I must warn you that your ward doctor has recommended that you be admitted into Sherrin here, for observation and wants a second opinion from myself. If my findings concur with his, he feels that it may then be necessary to transfer you to the mental health unit of Chelmsford Hospital. Do you understand?"

My heart was starting to pound and I could see Melanie looking at me with a worried expression on her face. The reality of my situation had finally dawned on me.

"Yes," I replied.

"Why did you secretly record two members of the hospital team, when they visited you in your home?" she asked.

"I don't know," I whispered.

"Your doctor told me that you thought they were attempting to get you admitted back into the hospital again. Is that correct?"

"I think so"

"You think that's what you told the doctor or think they were trying to get you re-admitted?"

"I can't remember"

She wrote something down on the clipboard on her lap and then said, "You were seen kissing a member of staff"

"Who said that?" I asked.

"Do you feel that you have a superiority complex and can manipulate female members of staff, until they succumb to your charm? Is that it?"

"No"

"On New Years Eve, you were reported vandalising the Christmas decorations in the hall and turning over the garden benches. Have you got a violent temper, John?"

Before I could think of anything to say, Melanie said, "John isn't a violent person. If anything, I'd say he was very caring"

The doctor glared at Melanie and said, "You are not a doctor and are not in a position to give a diagnosis. Please let John speak for himself"

"Melanie is right; I'm not a violent person. I'd just had my review that afternoon and was told that I had to stay for at least another three days"

"And because of that, you felt it was acceptable to cause damage to hospital property?"

"No…..I don't know. I thought I was going to be discharged and was really upset"

"Have you ever been violent towards your family? Towards your wife? Towards your children?"

"No I fucking haven't!" I yelled. "I would never hurt my kids in a million years!" and then I burst out crying.

Melanie held my arm and rubbed my back. The doctor looked at me without any emotion.

"Why are you getting upset, John?"

"I miss them so much!" I sobbed and buried my head in my hands.

"Do you have to do this right now?" asked Melanie but the doctor didn't reply.

After I'd calmed down, she said that she needed to make a phone call and would be back shortly. As she stood up, Melanie asked her, "Is it all right if John goes outside for a cigarette?"

The doctor looked over at the orderly and then said I could and she would call me when she had finished on the phone.

I followed Melanie outside and we walked over to a tree, where she hid behind the trunk.

"What are you doing?" I asked.

"I don't know about you but I need a fucking fag!" she said and offered me one.

"That bitch would do anything to try and get me out of here and I don't want her to see me smoking!"

I looked over towards the entrance to Sherrin and saw the orderly standing by the door, watching us. He looked at me and smiled.

"What is it with you and her?" I asked Melanie, "You're obviously not in her good books"

SECTION 3: LOW

"We had a riot in Cranbridge and she felt that I'd started it"
"Did you?" I asked and Melanie started to laugh.
"Well….yes but she didn't have any proof that I did"
"What happened?"
They treated us like criminals and we'd all had enough. I started smashing all the windows and setting light to the bed linen and then everyone joined in. You ask Zee, he was there"
"Did he join in with the riot as well?"
"He was only sixteen at the time and managed to break out. They found him about a mile away, hiding in the forest"
"Why were you in there Melanie?"
"It's a long story"
"Please tell me"
"My husband was a right bastard and used to hit me all the time. He thought I was having an affair," she said and burst out laughing. "Look at me; I'm not exactly the most glamorous woman on the planet, am I!"
I gave her a hug and replied, "I think you're brilliant!"
"I was in the launderette one Saturday afternoon and he came storming in, smelling of booze and knocked me out cold with one punch. I woke up in hospital with a broken jaw"
As she was telling me this, I could feel a rage burning up inside me. I wasn't a violent person but there was one thing I couldn't stand and that was a bully.
"Another time, he came in from work and started slapping me round the face in front of the kids. He then told them to stand in a row, ordered me to go to the end of the kitchen and forced them to watch as he

ran at me and kicked me in the shins with his steel toe cap boots"

"Why didn't you tell the police?"

"He said that if I ever did, he'd kill me and the kids"

"So how come you ended up being sectioned?"

"I lost the plot and tried to kill him with a bread knife. I ended up calling for an ambulance and they found me covered in blood, raving like a lunatic and saying over and over again that I was a bad person"

"What happened to him?"

"He survived, the cunt!"

"I'm so sorry Melanie," I said and gave her another hug.

"What have you got to be sorry for?"

"My problems seem like nothing, compared to what you've been through"

"You're wrong John; I saw how upset you were in there"

While we were talking, I had a text come through on my mobile and on opening it; I saw it was from Tina.

"I've just heard that you're in Sherrin Ward," it read, "What are you doing in there, is everything ok?"

I sent a text back to ask if she could talk and the next minute, my phone rang.

"John, what's going on? Davina just text me to say you're in Sherrin!"

"An independent doctor is assessing me and if it goes the wrong way, I'm in trouble"

"Where are you now?"

"Outside, having a fag with Melanie. I'm waiting for her to call me back in and give me the verdict. What about you, what happened with Victoria?"

"She was going to dismiss me but I resigned before she had the chance"

"You're joking!" I said, "What are you going to do?"
"I'll be okay. I should be able to get my old job back, giving home visits to elderly people"
"I feel terrible Tina, it's all my fault!"
"No it's not, it was my decision to kiss you and I'm glad I did but I'm worried about you John. If they keep you in Sherrin, then I may never see you again. I doubt if they'd let me visit you"
"Don't worry about me, I'll be alright. Where are you now?"
"I'm at Julie's, the hairdressers and she can't believe what's happening!"
She was starting to sound tearful and I tried to reassure her.
"Everything will be okay, you'll see. Tonight, we'll be laughing about this when you're round my place"
"That's why I was getting my hair done because I thought I was going to see you tonight but now I never will. I've always followed my head and not my heart but this time, I just don't know what to do?"
"Follow your heart," I replied.
Just then, the orderly called out for us to return to the assessment room.
"I've got to go Tina, they want me back inside"
"I'm so worried John"
"I'll speak to you soon," I said and hung up.
As we made our way over to the door, Melanie said, "You better hope it goes your way in there because if you end up in Chelmsford, you won't ever be right again"
Once we were back in the room, Melanie sat next to me again and she could see I was worried.
"Good luck," she whispered.

Doctor Jefferson walked into the room, followed by the crisis team and sat down opposite me.

"I've just been speaking to your ward doctor"

"SHIT!" I thought.

"I've recommended to him that you should not be re-admitted into hospital on the condition that you see the crisis team on a daily basis and do not attempt to record them again"

I gave an audible sigh of relief and noticed that my legs were shaking.

"Thank you," was all I could say.

"It's obvious to me that you have found it extremely difficult being separated from your children, since splitting up with your wife and have suffered a mental breakdown"

"You are the only person who's realised how much being away from my kids, has upset me," I replied and started to get upset again.

"You must also promise to take your medication. Even if you feel there is nothing wrong with you, the tablets will help to calm you down and think rationally"

"I promise to take them," I said and this time, I thought I meant it.

For three weeks, I had tried to 'fight the system' but now I was a broken man and realised finally, that I needed help.

"Your doctor said that if you agree to all of this, then he will agree with my diagnosis"

I wiped the tears from my eyes and thanked her again. She leant forward and placed her hand on top of mine.

"You can go now John and I hope you see your children soon"

SECTION 3: LOW

"I can't fucking believe it!" said Melanie when we were back outside. "I always thought she was a right cow but it turns out she has a heart after all!"
"Thanks Melanie, for being by my side"
"No offence John, I really like you but I don't ever want to see you here again"
"Don't worry mate, I've learnt my lesson"

I did return to the hospital though, for one last time, to see Melanie's colleague Claire. She'd told me she was a Pink Floyd fan and her favourite song was Comfortably Numb, off the album The Wall. I'd drawn a big picture relating to the lyrics of the song, back in 1987 and had it framed and decided to give it to her, so I went upstairs to their office and when she saw it, she loved it and was really grateful. She wanted it put up on the office wall but although I'd brought a picture hook with me, I'd forgotten to bring a hammer and so I went downstairs and then into the main hospital. Finding the maintenance room, I knocked on the door and when I asked to borrow a hammer, the guy didn't even question me.
After putting the picture up, I returned the hammer and said to the workman, "It's okay, I've wiped the blood off it!"
He looked at me suspiciously for a moment, so I winked at him and walked casually away down the corridor.

CHAPTER 38

I'd given Melanie a great big hug after she'd told me not to come back to the hospital again and then I got in my car and sent Tina a text, telling her that I was a free man! She rang me back straight away and said that she'd decided to leave her husband.
"Where are you?" I asked.
"I'm at home. He's just gone out to walk the dog and I'm going to tell him when he get's back"
"Give me your address," I said, "I'm coming round. I'm worried what he might do"
"He won't hurt me, if that's what you mean. I think he realises this was coming, anyway"
"I want to come just in case. Don't worry, I'll wait in the car, he won't know I'm there"
"Okay. Can I stay with you tonight John, until I find somewhere to live?"
"Of course you can, I want you to stay"
From the hospital, I drove straight round to Tina's and parked a few houses down. She looked out the window, saw my car and came to the front door. I flashed my headlights and she waved for me to get out the car and go over to her.
"He's still out walking the dog," she said.
"Have you got some stuff packed to bring to my place?"
"It's in the hallway. I'll put it in my car and come to you, after he's come back"

SECTION 3: LOW

At that moment, her husband appeared with the dog. There was an awkward silence for a moment and then I said, "I'm seeing Tina and she is moving in with me" He looked at me and then at Tina but said nothing and walked past her and went inside.
"Let me speak to him John and then I'll come round to yours," whispered Tina.

Back at my flat I waited for Tina to arrive but she didn't show. I eventually received a text message and it read: I won't be coming tonight. Need 2 sort a lot out. C u 2moro x
I felt like sending her a text back but decided it was best not to. While I was sitting there alone in the flat, I could actually start to feel my confidence disappearing and hated the fact that I was alone. You see in all these prison movies, where the inmate is finally released and he can't cope with the outside world. In prison, they are a somebody and have a place but outside, they are nobody. That's exactly how I was feeling and I'd only been in the hospital for three weeks. What must it be like for someone who'd spent years inside? I started to go through the mail and opened a letter from my wife's solicitor. It stated that I could see my daughter on the coming Saturday, for two hours in a church hall and under supervision. I would be able to see her once a fortnight under these conditions, until the foreseeable future. Two hours every two weeks! My own daughter and I had to be watched while I talked to her! It felt as if I were being treated like some sort of child molester or something and I can't tell you how angry and sick that made me feel. The only good part of it was that they had changed the meeting point to a nicer area, just a few miles away

from me. I wasn't even allowed to ring my wife, so I could speak to my daughter on the phone and it was driving me crazy. I felt absolutely helpless.

Tina arrived the following morning with some of her stuff and I was so pleased to see her. She said that she'd already contacted the company she'd worked for prior to the hospital position and they had arranged an interview with her for the next day. After she had unpacked her stuff, we went shopping for food and I'm not sure if it was my imagination but I could have sworn that everyone was staring at me. It was only a small village and everyone knew everyone's business. They must have all heard about me being sectioned and I hated it.
"I've got to get out of here," I told Tina.
"Why, what's the matter?"
"They're all looking at me and talking about me, I know they are"
"I can't see anyone looking"
"Please Tina, can you finish the shopping? I need to get back to the flat"
My phone rang when I got back and it was the crisis team, saying they wanted to see me in one hour but would not come to my flat (they didn't trust me after the recording incident) and had arranged to use one of the rooms at my local doctor's surgery. When Tina returned with the shopping, I told her about the call and she said that every time I was out of her sight, she was terrified that she'd never see me again. Tina thought that I would say the wrong thing and end up getting sectioned again.

I got to the doctors slightly early and told the lady behind the desk that I was waiting for the crisis team to see me and she asked me to take a seat. The waiting room was packed with pensioners, waiting to have their flu jabs and no sooner had I sat down than Saviour walked through the door with a lady I hadn't seen before. He saw me and nodded and then went over to the receptionist and said something. They then told me to follow them and all the pensioners looked at me as I stood up, wondering why I was being seen straight away and why I had two other people with me. I winked at this old lady sitting there and whispered, "It's okay, I get special treatment!"

We went down this corridor and into a doctor's room and he got up from his chair and asked Saviour if he could be as quick as possible as they were very busy. I apologised to the doctor and after he'd gone, I told Saviour that it wasn't right that all those people had to wait because of me. He said that they had to meet me there as I'd recorded them on their previous visit to my flat and so I promised that I'd never do it again.

"For the time being, we'll meet you here John"

"Well, what about at the hospital then?"

"Your ward doctor feels that you are a bad influence on some of the patients still being treated there and says that you like to make it known to them, when you are on hospital grounds"

I just shrugged my shoulders and sat down.

"Now then John........."

My mobile rang and it was Zee.

"Hey John you cunt, you're never gonna fuckin' believe it!"

"What?"

"They've only gone and discharged me, the fucking idiots! Ha ha ha ha ha ha ha ha ha ha ha!"
"Where are you now?"
"At the shopping centre. Can you pick me up and drop me round a mate's house, I'm fucking skint!"
"I'm a bit busy at the moment, ring me in a couple of hours and I'll come and get you"
"Alright boy, speak to you later!"
"A friend?" asked Saviour, after I'd hung up.
"Yeah….a good friend," I replied.
The meeting lasted for about twenty minutes, during which time I was asked if I had any suicidal thoughts.
"No," I answered.
"Have you seen Tina, since being discharged?"
"She's living with me"
Saviour looked at his colleague and then back at me.
"What are you trying to prove?" he asked.
"What do you mean?"
"Do you feel that you are somehow superior to us and can manipulate a member of the hospital staff?"
"I love her"
"And does she feel the same way about you?"
"I think so. She's left her husband and moved in to my place, so she must have strong feelings towards me"
"Would you be willing to allow us to speak to Tina in private?"
"What about?"
"We'd just like to hear her side of the story"
"It's not up to me, it's up to her"
"We have to ask your permission because it's you we are dealing with and she is your partner"
I could tell he struggled to use the word 'partner' and it was clear to me that they didn't take our relationship seriously.

SECTION 3: LOW

"If she wants to speak to you, then she can. I'll talk to her when I get back and let you know tomorrow," I explained.

When we walked back into the waiting room, Saviour spoke to the receptionist and arranged another appointment for the next day.

Back at the flat and Tina seemed relieved to see me.

"How did it go?" she asked.

"They want to speak to you"

"Why, what for?"

"They said they wanted to hear your side of the story"

"There's no way I'm going to speak to them, I know them all!"

"I told them I'd ask you but said it was up to you"

She went on for a while about not speaking to them and then started to get some pots and pans out of the cupboard.

"What are you doing?" I asked.

"Getting dinner ready for tonight. We've got spaghetti bolognaise"

"You don't have to cook for me, let me make you something"

"No, it's okay, I want to"

"Well if you insist. That reminds me, Zee rang me while I was in with the crisis team and he's been discharged"

"That's great news!"

"Yeh and I said that I'd pick him up later and bring him round for something to eat" (I just thought that last bit up on the spur of the moment)

I saw the look on Tina's face change and don't think she was too happy with the idea.

"I was going to cook for just us two, not Zee as well"

"Here we go," I thought to myself.

"I told you, I will do the cooking," I replied.
"No, no, I'll do it. I just wish you'd told me earlier about Zee"
"I only just found out a short while ago and anyway, what's the problem?"
"There's no problem, everything's fine"

While Tina got on with the spaghetti, I went to pick up Zee. I'd told him to wait by the taxi rank, outside the shopping mall and spotted him poncing a cigarette off a group of teenagers. I bibbed my hooter and he came running over to the car. It seemed strange seeing him out of the hospital ward, surrounded by 'normal' people.
"How you doing son?!" he bellowed as he slumped down into the car seat.
"Not bad mate, not bad"
"Thanks for picking me up, boy. What you been up to today?"
"I had to see the crisis team at my local doctors"
"I'm seeing them tomorrow at the hospital," he said, "how come you saw them at your doctors?"
I went on to tell him about the recording incident and how I'd told them that I couldn't afford the petrol money to go and see them and they'd have to come to me. He started to laugh and said, "You fucking nutter! I bet that really pissed them off"
"Just a bit"
When we got back to my flat, Tina was serving up our meal.
"All right Tina, how you doing darling?" boomed Zee and gave her a kiss on the cheek.
"I'm good thanks," she replied and looked like she was feeling awkward.

SECTION 3: LOW

I realised then, why she wasn't too keen on Zee coming round. She had been an orderly in the hospital where he had been a patient and now she was round my place, having dinner with him (and me, come to think of it)

Zee wolfed his food down and finished before me and Tina had hardly started.

"That was bleedin' gorgeous, I was fucking starving!" he said.

I offered him a beer and to my surprise, he declined.

"No thanks son, I can't with the meds I'm on. It makes me go a bit crazy" and then he started to have a go at all the doctors and nurses at the hospital and was becoming more and more irate.

I looked over to Tina and she gave me a look as if to say, "I think he had better go now" and so I told Zee that I'd take him to his mate's place.

"Yeh, yeh, no worries," he replied, "he's putting me up for a couple of nights but isn't supposed to have anyone else staying with him, so it's best I get there early so his landlord doesn't see me go in"

I felt a bit rotten, getting rid of him so quickly but he could be a bit of a lunatic. As I dropped him off at his friend's place, he gave me a hug and told me to thank Tina for the meal.

"I'll see you soon," I said.

"Yeh, I'll give you a ring," he replied and then he was gone. That was the last time I ever saw Zee.

The next day, Tina went for her interview and to her surprise, they gave her the old job back on the spot.

"I start on Monday," she said when she got back to the flat. "They've given me four homes to go to, all within two miles of this place"

I was really pleased for her but knew it meant she would be the only one earning any money. I just couldn't find it in myself to work and that's not me being lazy. Ask anyone who knows me and they will tell you that I've always worked really hard but since coming out of the hospital, my confidence had plummeted down to zero. In total, Tina and I lived together for only about six weeks. She was a brilliant person and I cared for her very much but something just didn't feel right. I started to realise that although I found her attractive, I was treating her as someone to look after me. I was seeing her as the Tina who worked on my hospital ward and not as a partner. It was by no means intentional and when I told her that I wasn't ready to go back to work yet, she told me not to worry and said that I had been unwell and it would take time.

CHAPTER 39

Saturday morning finally arrived and I was due to see my daughter at 10am, at the church hall. When I got inside, this lady told me to go over and sit by a table with a chair opposite it. I waited for about five minutes and then my daughter entered the room. She spotted me and came running over and I lifted her up and gave her the biggest hug ever. It was so great to see her.

We sat down at the table and I asked if she had a nice Christmas. She said that she missed me not being at home and felt sorry that I'd been unwell and in the hospital. I felt like crying my eyes out but managed to keep it together and we started to play some board games she'd brought with her.

I just didn't know what to say. I couldn't tell her that her dad had gone mad and ended up in a nuthouse! We drew a picture together and she asked if she could stay at my flat, one night.

"Soon," I answered.

I asked how the boys were and how she was doing at school and before I knew it, the two hours were up. I'd waited for what seemed like ages for that moment and it was over in a blink of an eye. The lady came over and told my daughter that it was time to go and I felt like telling her to fuck off! Who did she think she was, telling my little girl what she could and couldn't do! I gave her another big hug and said that I'd see her again in two weeks time and as she left the room, I started to cry. I didn't want anyone to see me upset and so to try and take my mind off it, I started to pack away the tables and chairs. Tears were running down my cheeks and I held my breath in for as long as I could. If I had started to breathe out, then I would have screamed out in agony. I couldn't look at anyone in the eye and just stared at the walls and floor. When all the tables and chairs had been put away, I started to head for the exit and the lady told me I couldn't leave yet.

"You're wife is outside, talking to my colleague and you can't leave until she has gone," she explained.

I was eventually allowed to go and when I got back to my flat, Tina was waiting for me. She could see I was upset and didn't say anything.

I started ranting and raving about only being allowed to see my daughter for such a short time and then I started crying again. I could feel such a pain within me and wanted to push my hands into my stomach and pull my insides out, thinking that would get rid of the awful feeling. Tina tried to comfort me but it was no use. I apologised to her and then went up to bed and cried and cried. The feeling of not being able to see my daughter was overwhelming and I could only imagine what it must have been like for someone who had lost a child. They would never be able to see them ever again and that thought began to haunt me. My mind was beginning to go into a dark place and I couldn't snap out of it. I'd been in the hospital for three weeks and only saw my daughter and youngest son once, for a short while and yet I'd been able to cope with it but now I'd been discharged, I was physically able to go and see my kids but wasn't allowed. It was driving me crazy and there were so many occasions when I wanted to get in my car and

SECTION 3: LOW

drive round to their house but I knew it would only make matters worse.

I'm finding this part of the book really difficult to write. For almost the entire next year, I felt totally depressed and just thinking back to that time is bringing my mood down considerably. I knew it would get to this stage and part of me wonders why I am putting myself through it but I feel that I have to get it out of my system by writing it all down.

This is the first thing I've written for about six weeks as I just couldn't face reliving the bad experiences over again and my mind came to a mental block.

In order to try and get myself back in the right mood and to try and remember what happened during this period, I requested for my medical records to be sent to me, hoping that would help. They arrived a couple of days ago, in a big white parcel and upon opening it; there was a brown envelope with a sticker on it reading in red ink:

CAUTION: Inside this envelope are the Medical Records you requested.

We recommend that you think carefully before opening the envelope as the contents may cause you some distress.

It may be sensible to read these notes in the company of your Advocate, CPN, a family member or friend.

Just reading that message alone made me appreciate that I had been through a traumatic experience but upon reading the notes themselves, I also realised how upsetting it all was for my family as well. I opened the envelope thinking there wasn't anything in there that I didn't know already and for the most part, I was right. I haven't found reading over my records to be distressing in any way but can imagine for some people that they could be very much so. Some of the patients in my ward had really gone through a terrible ordeal and I wouldn't recommend that some of them read their notes. I really hope they are better now (although for some of them, I doubt it) and think that to be reminded of what they had been through, would only do them more harm than good. I've always considered myself to be quite a caring person but since being sectioned and going through everything else that entails, I've realised I have become much more so. It's strange, just three weeks of my life was spent on that ward and yet it has had such a profound effect on me. I'll never forget my time spent there or all of the friends I made and it would make me so happy knowing, they were all well again. The main emotion I'm feeling reading over my records, isn't that of distress but more of embarrassment and shame. I'm embarrassed at the feelings of superiority when at the height of my bipolar, even though I know these are typical symptoms and ashamed at the way I spoke to my dad. I really don't know why I treated him so badly and didn't know until I read the notes, that he was totally against the idea of having me sectioned. Don't get me wrong, I can see now that it was the best and right thing for me but it must have been really hard for him to accept. I just have to keep telling myself over and over again that I was (am) mentally ill and it just wasn't me. It's a really difficult thing to say, "Mentally ill" but you have to accept it and deal with it, or you will never hope to live with it. I will get to it later but my dad died in December 2009 and although I apologised to him when he was in the hospital, I don't think I really meant it at that stage. It was terrible to see my dad ill but I was numb at the time, not just towards him but at everything and I think they were just words coming out of my mouth, to make him feel a bit better. I don't know if you can hear me dad but I really am sorry.

There was a part in the records that I really found interesting. There were copies of faxes sent between my G.P, the two psychiatrists and the social worker who came to see me at my sister's house, the night I was sectioned. Each fax had a date and the time it was sent and there were transcripts of telephone calls with my sister and also the police. It feels strange now that all that was going on and I didn't know anything about it. I mentioned earlier when I had been admitted into the hospital, I managed to keep my mobile phone on me and had tried to contact the two psychiatrists and the social worker, hoping to get them struck off (sorry about that, it seems ridiculous now)

I was speaking to my sister about this the other day and she said I'd called her and said, "I want those two doctors to get the sack and tell that social worker that I want her to clean my car!" (Total nutcase! Ha, ha)

In the notes, I found a record of a telephone call from the social worker to the hospital ward, expressing her concerns for her safety and wanting to know if I was still being detained. I must admit that when I read that,

BIPOLAR.....ME?

I had to smile just a bit. At the time, I hated her guts but had no intention of harming her and am sorry for any distress I caused her.

I've realised that you have to be so careful what you say as literally everything is noted down and sometimes, they aren't always accurate.

It makes me cringe to think that any doctor can look at these records and read that I claimed to have special powers and could smash glass, just by looking at it. My sister came to visit me at my flat before I was sectioned and I must have clearly been ranting and raving about something. I can remember telling her that my thoughts were so crystal clear, they could smash glass (not the cleverest thing to say, I must admit) but I didn't actually mean I had the power to break the glass with my thoughts. I was merely trying to describe how powerful those thoughts were.

That's what I mean about being careful what you say. The crystal clear thoughts rushing through my brain were obviously symptoms of the bipolar; it's just that I'd worded my feelings badly. I was trying to say that they were so intense; it felt as if they could smash glass but obviously it came out the wrong way. I don't know if my sister thought I'd meant I had special powers or when she told the doctors, they saw it that way but all I know is I didn't think I did. It all seems really silly now but if a doctor reads my records, he will always assume I thought I had this power and that just isn't the case. That time I thought I felt someone touch me on the shoulder when I was alone in my flat; I really did think that had happened and I admit it. I realise now that nobody touched my shoulder and it was probably due to lack of sleep combined with my illness but I definitely never thought I had special powers or was invincible. If I'd gone to the top of a tall building and jumped off or threw myself in front of a bus, I would have died….dead, finito. I may have been mad but I wasn't stupid. At the time, I had no suicidal thoughts whatsoever. I was feeling great and felt that I could do no wrong.

In the records, it states that I had feelings of superiority over others and in one way, I suppose that's the easiest way to describe it but it really isn't the case. It's more that I felt ultra confident and that was a really nice feeling, I just didn't behave in a sensible manner. There's no way I felt I was better than anybody else, it's more that I could see things they couldn't. I don't mean seeing things visually; more that I thought I'd discovered something, something that had taken away all my problems.

It's really hard to explain and put down into words. All I know now is that it was all a load of crap and how ridiculous I must have sounded. It's a good thing to be confident but when you start spending loads of money that you haven't got, then it's just fucking bonkers. I can see that now but when you are ill, you don't appreciate how it's going to affect you in the coming months and you don't care either. It's difficult knowing what is the right way to feel when you have bipolar and are finally taking the medication. For the most part, I'm feeling reasonably happy but as soon as I get in a really good mood, I start to question myself and wonder if this is normal behaviour. I find that I am constantly monitoring myself and how I am feeling but I suppose that's something I just have to live with. Scared isn't really the right word, more concerned that on the rare occasions I go out now for a drink with friends (I can't afford it much, I'm bleedin' skint!)

I might start losing the plot and go into a manic state again but as long as I keep taking the meds, then I suppose I will be okay.

Anyway, after reading through all of my records I was quite surprised at how much I remembered and have got right. It is awkward reading what the doctors have said about me but on the whole, I agree with everything they have recorded. That sounds like I am being arrogant and because I agree with them, then they were right after all. I don't mean it like that at all. At the time, I was convinced they had me all wrong but I now realise they knew exactly what was the matter with me. There is a bit in the notes that does make me sound arrogant though and that's when I said to the old lady in the doctor's waiting room, that I had special treatment. It's worded in such a way that says, John has bipolar therefore he has a superiority complex; therefore he feels he is more special than anybody else. I didn't mean it like that in the slightest and it's only because the crisis team don't know my sense of humour. It's the way everyone in the waiting room looked at me with surprise and annoyance. They had been waiting for ages to be seen when I waltzed in and not only was I seen straight away but also had two people to accompany me. I just said it as a joke and would love to have known what they were all thinking. If it had been up to me, I would have been the last person to have been seen and hated the fact that I'd jumped the queue. I mean, for heaven's sake, I am British after all! I suppose that's the only difficult bit. It's great feeling in a right state of mind again but at the same time, it can be quite hard reading all the truths about myself at the height of my bipolar.

CHAPTER 40

Sunday, 9am

I looked out of the window and everything was covered in thick snow.
"Here Tina, come and have a look at this"
She got out of bed and stood next to me.
"Oh no!" she said.
"What's the matter?"
"I've got to be up at half six tomorrow morning, to go to work"
It was the heaviest snow I'd seen in years and it was still coming down in big fucking lumps.
"Oh yeh," I replied, "still, we'll worry about that in the morning"
After breakfast, we decided to go for a walk but needed to get some wellies first and luckily for us, there was a shop open just across the road that sold them. When we opened the front door, Darren the window cleaner was standing there with a bucket in his hand.
"Do you want me to clean your car John?" he asked, with a big smile on his face.
"It's snowing, for fucks sake!" I replied. "Why don't you go home? You'll freeze to death!"
"They told me I should go out"
I could see Tina looking at me and introduced her. Darren smiled but I could tell he wasn't too happy. Before going into the hospital, Darren would often come round and I'd let him watch some of my DVD's

and make him something to eat. He'd obviously gotten used to the habit and could tell by Tina's presence, that it was all going to come to an end.

"Where are you going?" he asked.

"For a walk"

"Can I come?"

"No, sorry mate. We're going on our own"

I felt terrible saying that to him because I knew he was really lonely but I had to.

"Can I see you later John?"

"Er….. yeh. We're probably going down the pub, we might see you there"

Darren looked at Tina and then back to me.

"Okay John, I'll see you later then!" he said with a big grin and then turned around and trudged off through the snow with the bucket in his hand.

"Who was that?" asked Tina with a bemused look on her face.

"Darren"

"I know its Darren, you just told me but who is he?"

"Darren the window cleaner"

"Why did the window cleaner want to come for a walk with us?"

"Because I wouldn't let him clean my car"

"It's snowing like mad out there!" said Tina.

"I told him that but he'll be alright, he'll go and find some windows to clean"

"Are you sure he's a window cleaner?"

"Course he is, didn't you see the bucket?"

"He had the bucket so he could clean your car"

"That's his window cleaning bucket. What….do you think he has two buckets? One for cleaning windows and one for washing cars. Are you mad woman?"

"Me mad?"

"To be honest," I replied, "He's not the official village window cleaner. The real window cleaner can't stand him"
"Why's that?"
"Because when he's doing his rounds, cleaning the shop windows in the high street, Darren comes along afterwards and cleans them again"
"And the shopkeepers aren't prepared to pay twice?"
"It's not so much that, it's because he ends up leaving them in a worse state than before they were cleaned in the first place"
"What do the shopkeeper's do?"
"Most of them tell him to fuck off but he still carries on doing it, day after day. One woman has threatened to call the police"
"It's sad really," said Tina.
"He does okay. Some of the shopkeepers only use Darren and he makes enough to buy a couple of pints each night. The Indian uses him but they won't give him money, they pay him in curries instead"
"Oh well, are we going to go for this walk then or not?" she asked.
So we went across the street and bought our wellington boots and spent the morning walking through the fields surrounding the village. It stopped snowing for a while and the sun came out, turning the scene into something really beautiful. When we got back to the flat, we had some hot soup, snuggled up on the sofa and watched an old film on the telly (one of my DVD's I point out)
I was determined not to watch anything being broadcast!
"You're mad," said Tina.
"Well you did meet me in a mental hospital"

We went down the pub that evening and Wendy was serving behind the bar. There was no sign of Josh; I hadn't seen him since being discharged (which I was glad about because I knew he'd ask me about the comic and I felt so stupid)

I'd mentioned to Tina whilst in the hospital, about the tickets for the Nutcracker Suite and I asked Wendy if Bee still had them because I wanted them back. I figured that she hadn't once phoned me while I was in hospital to see how I was, so fuck her!

"Sorry John," replied Wendy, "she's ripped them up"

I just laughed and said, "Why did she do that?"

Wendy shook her head, "I don't know, the stupid girl. I don't know what's wrong with her"

I'd told Tina a few days earlier that I would get the tickets back and we could go instead. Wendy thought for a moment and then said, "All you have to do is ring them up and say the tickets didn't arrive. As long as you give them all your details, they'll send you some more"

"But it's on in two days time"

"If they send them by recorded delivery, you should get them by Tuesday morning"

"What, even with all this snow?"

"Well give it a go, it's worth a try," she replied.

We stayed in the pub for a couple of hours and upon returning to the flat, I rang the booking office and explained to them what Wendy had said. They told me not to worry and as long as I brought the same credit card along that I paid for the tickets with, they'd give us two more on the door.

"What happens if someone shows up on the night with the two original tickets?" I asked, "the postman might have taken them"

"We've made a note of it and will ask whoever arrives, to show us their credit card. If it doesn't match up to the payment on the tickets, they will not be permitted to enter"

"Oh, thank you so much….that's such a weight off my mind," I replied and winked at Tina, then hung up.

CHAPTER 41

Monday, 6:30am

Tina got up to take a shower. While she was in the bathroom, I got dressed, went downstairs and made us both a cup of tea.
"There's no need for you to get up," she said when walking out the bathroom and noticed the tea on the bedside cabinet.
"That's all right, I want to come with you," I replied, "besides, you might get stuck in the snow"
While Tina was getting dressed, I brushed my teeth and then we went downstairs for some breakfast. I looked out the window and it was still snowing heavily.
She had three houses to visit and we decided to go in my car. The snow was so heavy that you couldn't see where the road ended and the pavement began. All the kids were off school and instead of having a lie in; they were all out playing in the snow. I suppose Tina spent about twenty to thirty minutes in each house she visited and I had to leave the car running because it was so cold and I wanted the heater on. I remember while Tina was in one of the homes, I stared out of the windscreen and watched children making snowmen and having snowball fights and thought of my own kids.
"Where did it all go wrong?" I thought. "How did it get to this stage?"

SECTION 3: LOW

We eventually arrived back home at about 9am and as we pulled up outside, Darren was standing by the front door.

"Oh, not now," I said to Tina.

"Why don't you tell him to go away?" she replied.

"I don't know......... I can't"

We both got out of the car and I opened the front door.

"Hello John, hello Tina," said Darren.

Both of us smiled and nodded but said nothing and closed the door, leaving him standing outside.

"I can't live here anymore Tina," I whispered.

"Why, what do you mean?"

"Every time I open the door, he's there and it's not just him. When I walk out of here, it's straight into the main road and everyone's looking at me. They know what's happened to me, they know where I've been!"

"I thought you loved it here," she replied.

"I do. I love the flat and I used to love its location but now I feel that every time someone walks past, they're talking about me"

At that moment, there was a squeaking noise and I realised that Darren was washing the window. I walked over to it and pulled the blind down.

I had to get out. It felt like a huge weight was piling up on top of me.

"I must admit," said Tina, "we could do with some more space, I've got nowhere to put my clothes"

"Before I was sectioned, I viewed a two bedroom flat just along the road," I explained. "We could rent that and put some wardrobes in the spare bedroom, that way we'll have plenty of space"

"But I thought you said you didn't like the location"

"I like the village, it's not having the privacy....this is different. We could rent a flat on the second floor and there's an intercom system, so no one could come up without us letting them in the main door on the ground floor"

In hindsight, maybe we should have moved out of the village all together. Everyone knew everybody else's business and I was becoming increasingly paranoid that they were all talking about me, behind my back.

"How much is the rent," asked Tina.

"I don't know but I did look into buying one" (I thought it best not to mention that I'd actually considered buying the whole building without a penny to my name!)

"We can't afford to do that"

"I realise that but I know the owner, his office is just across the street. We can go and ask him and you can have a look at the place"

So that's what we did and Tina really liked the flat. When we got home, we talked about it for a while and decided to go for it. My flat was furnished but this one wasn't, so that meant we'd have to fork out for a bed, sofa, wardrobes and dining table etc. It had a fully fitted kitchen with dishwasher, washing machine / tumble dryer but nothing else (apart from the bathroom suite)

The rent was £900 a month and I phoned the guy back and offered £800.

Because the global economy was in such a sorry state, property just wasn't shifting and we figured that he'd be only too happy to have someone in one of his properties. The receptionist answered and explained he wasn't in his office but said she'd give him the message and get back to me.

SECTION 3: LOW

Tuesday

After I'd taken Tina to make her house visits, we drove to the supermarket to do some food shopping. It had finally stopped snowing the previous night but now the roads were icy and there were crashed cars all over the place. While we were at the check out, my phone rang and it was the guy who owned the flats. He said he was prepared to accept £850 a month but I stuck to my guns and he finally agreed to the £800. I told Tina and we were both in good spirits, which set us up nicely for seeing the Nutcracker, later that evening. Back at the flat, we started unloading the shopping and my phone rang again. The crisis team wanted to see me in one hour at the doctor's surgery and asked again, if Tina would come but when I told her, she was adamant that she wasn't going. I went on my own to see them and it was all the usual crap but I really respected the team because it was obvious, they only had my best interests at heart. When I got back to the flat, we both got dressed up really smart and went down the pub for a quick drink (well, we had to start the evening off on the right footing, didn't we?)

I told Wendy that we could pick the tickets up when we got there and she told us to have a really good time. I don't know if it was my imagination but I felt that Wendy was feeling guilty about Bee ripping up the tickets. I don't know why, it wasn't her fault. Maybe it was her daughter Zoe, who'd told Bee to do it? Tina drove us to the nearest station and when we got to Covent Garden, we found this pub that looked rather inviting and consumed several beverages. Afterwards, we had a walk round and found this Italian restaurant and decided to go in for a meal. I had three Peroni's and Tina, white wine……oh….and some food of course. When we finally got to the Royal Opera House, we went to the booking office and sure enough, they had our tickets waiting for us. I reminded them that, if the postman / lady turned up, meaning Bee or a friend of hers (I had this feeling she was going to try and use them) then not to let them in. They told me not to worry and if someone did try to use the original tickets. they would be ejected from the premises. Part of me hoped that Bee would turn up and try and get in, I would have loved to have seen her get slung out.

Anyway, we were a bit early and so made our way to the bar for some more refreshments. About half an hour later, the bell rang as a signal we had to go and take our seats and we were right down on the front row.

They were by no means the most expensive seats because we overlooked the orchestra pit but for me, that was a bonus. I loved watching the musicians play while the ballet dancers performed on stage and found it fascinating, listening to not just the music but the noises made when people were supposed to be creeping along or doors opening etc. These were the things you would usually take for granted and not be aware it was in fact the orchestra creating those sounds. The costumes and sets were magnificent and I was totally caught up in the whole thing. All in all, we had a brilliant day and what made it better was, Tina didn't have to work the next morning, so we didn't need to get up early.

Over the next few days, it started to warm up and the snow slowly melted away. We spent that time looking for furniture but part of me wasn't the slightest bit interested. I found that I was on autopilot and just went along with the flow, pretending to be excited and looking forward to us moving in on the following Monday. Tina couldn't wait though and I think there was part of me thinking, "I've just come out of a relationship and now I'm going straight into another one"

I didn't know what I wanted to be honest. One minute I was feeling good and the next, incredibly low but I didn't want Tina to become concerned.

She was such a great person, who obviously had a lot of feelings for me and I just wanted to see her happy. Looking back now, I should have told her I didn't want to go ahead with it and even had doubts about us being together in the first place but I just couldn't do it. What was wrong with me? Happy, low, happy, low, happy low……..low, low….low.

When I was discharged, I couldn't stand the thought of being on my own and yet now, that's exactly what I wanted.

Was that what I wanted? I thought it was but I really didn't know. I felt like screaming.

Looking back to that time, I can see now that my bipolar was turning from a massive high and starting to spiral downwards. On the Friday, Tina had to go out in the afternoon to do her house visits and I stayed at home. I was feeling really bitter towards my family and especially my dad (I wrongly thought he had a big part in getting me sectioned) and I'd been phoning him constantly, just to insult him basically. I rang my mum and dad's number and when my mum answered, I asked if dad was there.

"Why do you want him John?" she replied and thinking about it now, I could hear the anguish in her voice and the concern in my dad's voice in the background. I feel so ashamed now. Even if my dad had played a part in getting me sectioned, it was for my own good. My brother had told me previously to stop bothering them, as they were not young anymore and I was really upsetting them but I took no notice. My mum eventually passed the phone over to my dad.

"Are you all right John?" he asked.

"Don't fucking pretend that you care!" I yelled, "I can't stand you!"

"If that's the way you feel John, why do you keep on ringing me?"

"When you die, I'm going to piss on your grave!"

He hung up on me.

Now anyone who knows me will tell you that just wasn't me. I'm not a malicious person in the slightest and wouldn't want harm to come to anyone.

It was such a terrible thing to say.

I've thought a great deal about whether I should include what I said to my dad in the book because I'm so ashamed but have come to the conclusion that I must. I was listening to the radio the other day and they were talking about all these horror films coming out lately, dealing with exorcisms and possession. They said that in real life, the most obvious answer for the apparent symptoms of possession is mental illness, which I totally agree with. They then played a piece of recording someone had done on their mobile phone, of an air stewardess on a plane in America that was just about to take off. She had suddenly got out of her seat and ran down the aisle, screaming in a really eerie way. Everyone who heard her said that it sounded like

something out of the Exorcist and she appeared to be possessed but when I listened to it, all I could hear was somebody screaming out in fear. To me, she'd had some sort of mental breakdown and the part of her brain that said she was scared of flying (which had obviously been deeply hidden) suddenly came to the fore. I heard exactly the same screams when I was in the hospital. So maybe there was a part of my brain that had malicious thoughts, buried deep just like the fear of flying was buried deep inside the mind of the air stewardess?
I don't know.
That's how I think of what I said to my dad. The easiest way to describe it was that I sounded possessed.

My hope is that other people suffering from bipolar disorder will read this because only they will truly know what I was going through. I'm sure it affects people in all different ways but basically, when it comes down to the bare bones of the illness, it's all the same. There are plenty of famous people that suffer with my condition and I can understand that entirely. It must be so easy to get grandiose feelings when people adore you and also, be terribly depressing because you can never live up to people's expectations of you. I've mentioned before that I'm useless with money. To suddenly become wealthy, would probably be the worse thing that could happen to me. I had been so convinced that my website idea was going to become an enormous success but just say it had, I would have gone totally off the rails and who knows what would have happened to me?

So my dad hung up and I immediately rang him back. No answer. I rang again, no answer. I then found the telephone number for my mum and dad's local police station and called them. When they answered, I explained that my parents were quite elderly and didn't go out much.

"I know they are at home," I said, "but nobody is answering the phone and I'm really worried. Could you send someone round to check up on them?"

Why did I do that? I really don't know.

To this day, I still don't know if the police did actually go round and check up on them. I'm too ashamed to ask my mum and just wished it had never happened in the first place.

CHAPTER 42

Saturday, 8am

I'd initially been told via my wife's solicitor, that I could see my daughter once a week, on a Saturday morning but then discovered that it was actually, once a fortnight. That news absolutely devastated me and because this was the Saturday I would not be seeing her, my mood was rock bottom to say the least. Tina knew how I was feeling and tried to comfort me the best she could.
"Some of the furniture is being delivered this morning," she said, "we could go over to the flat and you can put it together"
"Fucking great!" I thought to myself but tried to look enthusiastic.
The landlord / owner of the flats had agreed that we could start moving furniture in before we officially moved in on the Monday.
I received a call from the delivery people and met them over at the new flat and helped take the boxes up the two flights of stairs to the second floor and dump them all in the middle of the living room.
"I am _so_ not in the mood for this," I thought to myself.
Tina said she was going out to get towels and all that malarkey and did I want to come?
"That's okay, I'd better start getting this stuff made up," I replied.

I just wanted to be on my own and the last thing I needed was to be walking around the shops, looking at fucking curtains and things!
"Isn't it exciting!" she said as she walked out the door.
"Yeah, triffick," I whispered under my breath.

When I say that my old flat was furnished, it was in fact only partly furnished. It had a double bed, a dining table and chairs and a coffee table. My youngest son's mate gave me his wardrobe and bedside cabinets and chest of drawers because his mum and dad were doing his bedroom up and buying him a load of new stuff. The only thing I had to buy was a sofa-bed, which I got off some woman on eBay. My thinking at the time was to get a sofa come bed, in case my kids or friends came over to stay. Tina and I had ordered a new sofa-bed because mine was on its last legs, after my nephew had half demolished it the time he stayed the night but it wasn't due to be delivered for a couple of weeks, so we had to use my old one in the meantime. The normal bed was being delivered on the Monday (moving in day) and a new wardrobe, a couple of days later. The plan was to put my furniture in the spare bedroom and I'd keep my clothes in there while Tina could bung all her stuff in the new wardrobe.

Over the years, Tina's kids had bought her these collectable fairy things that you put in a display cabinet but she'd never gotten round to actually take them out of their boxes. I'd promised her we'd get a display cabinet and she could finally have them on show. Tina said it didn't really matter but I knew she was very fond of them and I thought they were nice too.

SECTION 3: LOW

So when she went out to get the frilly curtains and towels, I was determined to assemble the display cabinet first and get all of the fairies in it before she got back. Even though I was feeling depressed, I really wanted to make her happy and thought it would be a nice surprise. I know there will be people reading this thinking, "That was totally wrong, what she did. She should never have gotten into a relationship with a patient," and you'd be absolutely right but Tina didn't have one bad bone in her body.

Her married life was obviously in a right state (although when she had been working on the ward, you would never have known it)

She had this natural ability to lift everyone's spirits when she came on to do her shifts and had such a friendly and caring way about her. When Zee and Dominic found out we were having this thing going on together in the hospital, they both told me to look after her and not hurt her feelings. She had that effect on people, she was so naturally caring that people felt caring towards her.

When I'd started flirting with her on the ward, I didn't know it would end up how it did. I suppose I wanted to be loved and over the course of time, I could tell that she had genuine feelings for me. You've got to understand that at the time, I was this ultra confident person who couldn't do anything wrong. I don't mean that in a big-headed way because I can't stand people who think about themselves that way but I just seemed to have this natural charm that rubbed off on people. After I'd seen my wife, second son and daughter in the hospital, with Tina present in the room, she told me the next day that she thought my wife would have been some blonde bimbo type, like a footballer's wife.

"No way!" I said, "That's not my cup of tea"
"She seems lovely," replied Tina, "why did you split up?"
"It's a long story, she's a great person and very caring. We just grew apart, that's all"
That's when Tina started to tell me about her marriage and how unhappy she was, so in her defence, all I can say is she wasn't thinking straight when she said she wanted to go out with me.

I finally got the display cabinet finished and fitted a light inside, then arrange all of the fairies out on the glass shelves, just in time before Tina came back from the shops. She was so thrilled to see them on display and her reaction lifted my mood considerably.
"Shall we go home now?" I asked, "And I'll finish making the rest of this stuff up tomorrow"
"Yes, of course but let me show you what I've bought first!"
"Oh, okay!" (Mood starting to drop down again)
I pretended to be interested in all the stuff she'd bought and then we fucked off back home.

Sunday.
Tina was at my place, packing up bits and pieces while I was putting the rest of the furniture together in the new flat. I could feel the weight of depression getting heavier on top of me and seemed to be moving in slow motion. What would normally take me about thirty minutes to put together, was now taking over two hours. Every so often I would stop what I was doing and burst out crying for seemingly no reason but eventually got two pieces of furniture assembled, when my phone rang.

SECTION 3: LOW

"How you getting on?" asked Tina.

"Slowly," I mumbled.

"Why don't you call it a day and come back? You can do some more tomorrow"

"I'll be home soon; I just want to finish the one I'm working on"

In reality, I couldn't face being with anyone and spent the next half an hour sitting on the floor, surrounded by cardboard boxes and bits of furniture, crying. When I finally got back home, I saw that Tina had managed to pack up quite a lot of stuff and was now cooking dinner. I remember trying my hardest to put on a front and pretend I was feeling good but I don't know if she could tell I wasn't. After we'd eaten, Tina had to go out and do some home visits and once I'd done the washing up, I started to take down all of the film photos I had stuck up all over the walls. When I'd first put them up, I used white Blu Tack because I didn't want to leave any marks on the walls when it came to removing them. I figured that the landlord might use some of my deposit to have the walls repainted if necessary but it was unlikely though because he was such a nice bloke. When my cousin Lee had picked me up from the hospital (the first time I was discharged) he was driving me to my mum and dad's and had to stop for petrol. My phone rang and it was my landlord sounding worried.

"John, are you okay? I haven't seen you for a while," he said.

"Yeh, yeh, I'm fine. I've just spent a few days with my mum and dad," I lied.

"I hope you don't mind but I went inside your flat, to check everything was all right. Everyone's been asking where you are"

"Nah, that's all right mate. I'll be back this afternoon, I'll see you later"
After I'd hung up, Lee said, "That's nice innit. He seems like a really nice fella"
And he was. When I told him I was moving out before the end of my agreed six month lease, he said it was fine as long as someone else rented it when I left. I already knew a couple who were interested, so that was no problem. Even with that being the case, I removed the photos as carefully as possible and slowly rolled the White Tack off the walls but could see that it was still leaving a mark. It wasn't a coloured mark, more of an oil stain from whatever the stuff was made of. You might think, "So what. What's the big deal?" but there were hundreds of photos all over the place and with four bits of White Tack for each photo, the walls looked terrible!
I knew the guy who'd decorated my flat when it had been built. He was a regular down Wendy and Duncan's pub and had moved to England about ten years earlier, from Northern Ireland. Wendy hated him and told me he was a complete bullshitter and after speaking to him for five minutes, I had to agree with her. He told me that he was a member of the IRA and also a part time stand-up comedian as well as a painter decorator. I'm sure what most of he was telling me was true (you couldn't make it up) but you could tell he was exaggerating a lot. Every time you'd go into the pub, he'd tell you one of his jokes and at first it was funny but after a while, you just felt like telling him to fuck off. He had this hobby of collecting all things concerning Egyptian Pharaohs and went out there a couple of times a year. That's believable but when he went on to say he was best mates with the

SECTION 3: LOW

curator of The Museum of Egyptian Antiquities and he allowed him to look at all these artefacts that the general public weren't allowed to see, one began to question the validity of his Egyptian fable. He was a nice enough bloke really and was always friendly towards me. Anyway, I decided to see him first thing in the morning and ask if he still had any of the paint left, he'd used to decorate the flat. When Tina got in, we pulled out the sofa-bed, perched a load of lit candles on top of the boxes she'd packed, turned off the lights and snuggled up to watch an old movie.

Monday morning and Darren was cleaning the window downstairs.
Tina had already gone off to work so I made Darren a cup of tea, said good morning and noticed the decorator across the road, loading up his van. I ran across to see him and asked if he had any of the paint left.
Luckily he said he did and gave it to me and lent me a paint brush.
I spent the next two hours painting over the marks on the walls, while Darren made me copious cups of tea. When Tina got back, she went over to see the landlord of the new flat to finalise the paperwork and got an extra set of keys. The flat was literally a two minute walk away and I asked Darren if he could give me a hand to take my furniture over to the new place.
Carrying the wardrobe with one person at each end, you would expect the journey to take about five minutes but with Darren's help (bless him) it took over half an hour, with us going all over the place. Passers-by were being scattered left, right and centre as Darren huffed and puffed and almost kept dropping

the fucking thing. At one point, he walked backwards into the road (I started off from the flat walking backwards but somehow we ended up swapping around) and nearly got run over. Cars had to swerve out of the way and they bibbed their horns in anger. I wouldn't have minded but he was carrying <u>my</u> wardrobe! We eventually got to the entrance door of the new block of flats and Tina had already propped it open for us but it was obvious we weren't going to get the wardrobe up the stairs, without taking it apart. The problem was as soon as you went through the door, the floor area was only big enough to let the door swing back against the wall. Once inside, the stairs were immediately on the right and led up to the first floor. Before we even got inside the entrance, it was clear to me that it wasn't going to work and so I told Darren to stop but he ignored me and pulled the wardrobe through the doorway, with me still hanging on to the other end. The wardrobe was now wedged inside this tiny space, with Darren's legs trapped underneath it and the rest of him sprawled up the stairs.

"Fucking marvellous!"

"Having trouble?" called out Tina and peering my head around the doorway, I could see her standing on the stairs, just above Darren's crumpled body.

"HELP ME, HELP ME!" yelled Darren, "I'm stuck!"

I was unable do anything because I just couldn't fit through the doorway and so Tina crouched down, put her hands under Darren's armpits and started to pull.

"AAAARRRRRGGGGGGGHHH! HELP ME, HELP!" cried the useless lump.

"That ain't gonna fucking work!" I said, "he's stuck fast!"

SECTION 3: LOW

It was like a bleedin' Laurel and Hardy sketch and Tina was in fits of laughter.

"Well, what do you suggest?" she asked.

"I'll run back to the flat and get a screwdriver. I'll have to take it apart before we can shift that dozy fucker!"

So I made my way back to the old flat and could hear Tina oofing and arring and Darren yelling, "HELP ME!" over and over again.

When I got back, Tina had obviously managed to pull Darren out from under the wardrobe because he was now inside it, tearing the doors off with his bear hands. I just about heard Tina saying, "I don't think you should be doing that" but he was oblivious and just carried on.

"What the fuck are you doing?" I yelled.

"I'm taking it apart for you," replied Darren with a look of pride on his face.

"You're fucking ruining it, you idiot!"

"It's all right John, I've nearly done it!"

"Get the fuck out of there now!"

He took no notice of me whatsoever and so I had to literally drag him out of the wardrobe.

"Is there anything wrong John?" he asked.

"RUINED! LOOK AT IT! FUCKING RUINED!"

The hinges on the doors had been torn out of the sides of the wardrobe with wild abandon and made big holes in the chipboard.

"Once we get this upstairs, I'll give you a hand with the rest of the stuff," said Darren politely.

"FUCK OFF!"

"Don't you want me to help you anymore?"

"NO! NOW GET OUT OF MY FUCKING SITE!"

"Oh, okay John. I'll be back later and I'll clean your windows for you"
"They're already clean you idiot and how you gonna reach? I ain't letting you inside you hear me…..EVER!"
"That doesn't matter," he replied, "I've bought this extending pole especially, so I can reach!"
"GET AWAY FROM ME!"
"But John…."
"FUCK OFF!"
With that, Darren walked up the road whistling to himself and called out, "Bye John. I'll see you later!"

Between us, me and Tina managed to get the wardrobe apart, carry it upstairs and put it back together in the spare room. Luckily, the side with the holes in it went up against a wall and didn't show. All I had to do was reposition the hinges and it was back to normal (almost)

It took about an hour and a half to get everything else from the other flat and when we eventually got the sofa-bed into the living room, we slumped down in it, knackered.

Both of us were drained and sat there in silence for a few minutes until finally, Tina turned to me and said, "What's that noise?"

We both looked over to the window and could see a pole with a lump of old rag stuck on the end of it, smearing the glass with muddy water.

"OH, FOR FUCK'S SAKE!"

CHAPTER 42

Tuesday.

After waking up on the bedroom floor (we were waiting for the bed to be delivered sometime that day) Tina got ready and went off to work and I stayed at home in case the bed came while we were both out. I made myself a cup of tea and had a couple of cigarettes on the balcony, before going into the spare bedroom and unpacking some of my things. We'd bought a CD shelf holder a few days previously and my plan was to put it together and then stack the shelves. It was a bit tight for space trying to construct the thing in the bedroom but I finally got it completed and then opened one of the boxes containing my CD's. On top of all the disk cases was a school photo of my daughter and I took it in my hands and stared at her face.
God, I missed her so much!
I had to stop what I was doing and went and made myself another cup of tea and had several more cigarettes. My mood dropped considerably and I really wasn't in the right frame of mind to continue unpacking the CD's and so decided to have a bath instead. For some reason, I felt that I needed to be wrapped in warmth of some kind (I wasn't cold and the flat was well heated)
It's hard to explain but I knew if we'd had the bed already, then I would have been underneath the duvet feeling safe. Once the bath had run, I climbed in and

pulled my knees up under my chin and burst out crying. Staring up at the bathroom ceiling, I could see an image of my two boys when they were five and three years old in their pyjamas and blue dressing gowns, the ones with the ladybird buttons. They were standing by the Christmas tree, hugging each other and I was filming them with my dad's video camera. After I'd transferred the tape onto a normal sized video cassette, I dubbed over it with John Lennon's Happy Xmas (War Is Over) and I just couldn't get that image and that song out of my mind. I buried my face into my knees and spent the next half an hour sobbing.

After I climbed out of the bath and got dressed, I went back into the spare bedroom and picked up the photo of my daughter again. I knelt down on the floor and just stared at it for ages, crying my eyes out. Tina opened the front door and saw me in the bedroom and asked if I was okay but I still couldn't take my eyes off the image of my daughter's face. When I didn't answer her, Tina walked into the kitchen and I could hear her put the kettle on. It took about another ten minutes before I calmed myself down and then I joined her in the living room, sitting down next to her on the sofa.
"I bet you've got second thoughts now?" I said and gave a forced laugh but she didn't reply and put her hand on my leg in a reassuring way.
My mobile phone started to ring but I just sat there.
"Aren't you going to get that?" asked Tina and I eventually got up and answered the phone.
"Hello"
"Hello John, this is Saviour from the crisis team. Can we meet you at the doctor's surgery in one hour?"

SECTION 3: LOW

"Yes," I replied and hung up.
"The crisis team?" asked Tina.
"Yeh"
"You should tell them how you're feeling John"
"I will….I promise"
So I went to the doctor's surgery and even before I said anything, Saviour could tell I was feeling low. I explained that I was missing my kids and he said that everything would work out in the end. That didn't make me feel much better to be honest because when was the end? He asked if I was still taking the medication and I lied that I was. Even though I had promised the doctor at my assessment in Sherrin ward that I would take the meds, I still wasn't (and looking back now, I've no idea why)
Because Tina had worked at the hospital, I figured she would be checking that I had been taking them, so I would take one out each morning, wrap it in toilet paper and flush it down the loo and do the same thing each evening. If she looked in the packet, she'd see that the tablets were being removed at the right time each day and therefore assume I had been taking them. Again, the crisis team asked me if Tina would come the next time and again, I said that I'd ask her. When I got back to the flat, I was feeling a little bit better and apologised to Tina for being a miserable git! She told me not to be silly and we sat on the sofa for the next hour, holding each other close. She said that she still didn't want to see the crisis team and I replied, "fair enough"
The bed finally arrived at about five in the afternoon and after helping the blokes lug it up the stairs; I put it together while Tina made us something to eat. Our bedroom had a skylight in it which was situated

directly above the bed and I remember saying to Tina before we moved into the flat, how great it would be that we could lie there and look at the stars. That night after Tina had fallen asleep, I lay on my back staring out of the skylight and felt totally and utterly miserable. I'm so sorry Tina; you had done absolutely nothing wrong. I could actually feel myself getting more and more depressed by the second and just hoped that everything would be all right in the morning.

Wednesday, 6:30am.
I was woken by the sound of Tina getting out of bed and immediately realised that everything was not all right. Lying on my side with my back to her, I pretended to still be asleep and was grateful that she got ready and left without trying to wake me. I desperately didn't want her to see me like I was the day before and was determined to try and snap out of it before she came back from work. As soon as the front door closed, I got out of bed and had a shower, figuring that because I'd got so upset in the bath the previous morning, a shower would somehow make it all okay. I suppose it helped slightly but I wouldn't say I was jumping for joy! I'd suffered from depression in the past and so recognised the signs of its onset but knew that it was going to be a lot worse this time. Tina only had a couple of houses to visit that morning and was back within the hour.
"I've got to go out again after lunch," she said, "to see three more people"
"I'll come with you and wait in the car," I replied.
"Are you sure?"

"Definitely!" (Anything to try and change the way I was feeling)

So after lunch, I drove Tina to do her rounds and the last house was in this small cul-de-sac. It was about half way down and as I waited for Tina, another car pulled up behind me with two women in it. Looking in my rear-view mirror, I could see that they were talking and still hadn't got out the car but I took no notice and waved to Tina as she came out the house.

"Everything okay?" I asked as she got in the car.

"Yeh," she replied, "he's a really nice man and hardly ever sees anyone all day............. OH FUCK!"

"What's the matter?"

"Look, its Victoria!" she said.

I looked out of the windscreen and saw Nurse Ratched and a young nurse from my ward, walking past us to the end of the cul-de-sac.

"Get down!" said Tina and we both crouched down in our seats.

I peered through the steering wheel and could see them ringing the doorbell of a house at the bottom of the street.

"It's all right," I whispered (I don't know why, they couldn't have heard me anyway) "they've gone inside one of the houses"

"Quick, let's get out of here!" said Tina and we both sat upright again.

As I started to reverse out of the cul-de-sac, another car turned into the road and instead of backing out of the way, the bloke just sat there.

"Oh no!" yelled Tina and when I looked forward, I could see Victoria and the nurse walking back down the street.

"That was a fucking quick house call!" I said.
"Maybe the person didn't want to see them?"
The man in the car behind started bibbing his hooter and it was clear that he wasn't going to shift.
"I'll have to drive to the end of the road and turn round," I explained to Tina.
"But we'll go straight past them and they'll see us!"
"I think they already have," I replied.
Victoria was staring straight at us and she didn't appear to be too happy. Me and Tina looked at each other pretending to be in deep conversation, so it seemed that we hadn't noticed her and the man in the car started bibbing again. I hit the accelerator and we whizzed past Victoria and the nurse like a shot. Talk about trying to be inconspicuous. After turning around at the dead end, I drove back up the road, only to be confronted by the bloke who'd been bibbing his hooter, reversing his car into the spot we'd been parked in. It was taking him ages to get the car in the space and Victoria sat glaring at us through her windscreen, so I slowly squeezed through the gap between his car and the vehicle parked on the other side of the road. As we passed Victoria and the nurse, all four of us looked at each other awkwardly as the sound of swearing came from the irate man in the other car. We couldn't stop laughing all the way back to the flat but because I was depressed, it was more like a nervous laugh and somehow seemed the wrong thing to do.

Back home and I could feel my mouth turning down at the sides and it felt so comfortable and natural. That sounds really strange I know but to actually physically smile, felt like it would take a monumental effort. We ate our evening meal in silence (at least, I was silent)

SECTION 3: LOW

Tina tried to cheer me up by talking about the Victoria incident but it was clear that it wasn't working. I just stared down at my food and pushed it around the plate with my fork, too ashamed to look up and stare her in the face. She went out at six that night, to do a couple of more rounds and as soon as she'd gone, I went straight to bed. I wasn't in the least bit tired, more that I needed the comfort of the duvet around me as if it would somehow protect me and make me feel better. I must have dozed off at some point and was woken by the sound of the front door closing. Tina called my name and then gently pushed open the bedroom door. I just couldn't face seeing her because I was so incredibly low and so I pretended to be asleep again. I heard her sigh and then shut the door, leaving me on my own in the darkness.

Thursday, 10am.
Tina had come back from work to find me sitting on the sofa with my head in my hands. It's funny but before going through such a deep depression, I would not have understood at all and just told that person on the sofa, to buck their ideas up. Even now, writing about it, I must sound like such a pathetic person but there was absolutely nothing I could do to stop myself feeling that way. Tina's mobile rang and after speaking on it for a short while, she hung up and said, "I don't fucking believe it, the wardrobes aren't coming now for a couple of weeks!"
She never lost her temper and I knew it must have been because of me. I looked at her and tried to give a reassuring smile but I very much doubt if it came across that way. My phone rang and it was the crisis team again, asking to meet me in an hour.

"I'm going with you!" said Tina after I'd hung up.
"But I thought you said…."
"I know but I think it's best I should"
When we got to the surgery and inside the doctor's room, I could sense the awkwardness because Tina knew all of these people professionally. Saviour asked her how she was keeping and she replied that she wasn't too bad.
"I hope you don't mind John," he said to me, "but I'm going to ask Tina some questions concerning you"
I shook my head and said that I didn't mind.
"You can go to the waiting room if you'd prefer not to be present," he continued. I looked at Tina and she said that she'd rather I heard what she had to say.
"John is very depressed," she said, "and I think the main reason is due to the fact that he has limited time to see his children"
"Are you and your wife trying to resolve the situation?" he asked me.
"Well, our solicitors are," I replied.
"Are you still taking your medication John?"
"Yes"
Saviour then turned to Tina and gave a look as if to ask the same question. "Oh shit!" I thought, "What if she knows?"
"Yes he is," she said. "I hope you don't mind John but I checked because I was worried about you"
Phew!
I held her hand and said, "Of course I don't mind"
Saviour reiterated that things would slowly get easier and after going on for a while about me continuing to take the meds, we left and went back home.
"I'm sorry John," said Tina back at the flat.

SECTION 3: LOW

"Don't be," I replied, "I should be the one apologising to you"
My mum rang early in the evening to ask if her and Pauline could come and visit me on the Saturday. I explained that I was due to see my daughter at the church hall at ten in the morning for two hours but could meet them after I came out. She said that would be fine and asked me how I was and I played down how low I was really feeling. The thought of seeing my daughter soon, lifted my spirits some what and Tina and I had a nice evening for once. I could just tell that she regretted getting involved with me because she'd told me that she had absolutely loved her job and must have realised the mistake she'd made. I had been sectioned and diagnosed with bipolar disorder and when I was in the hospital, I was still on a high. Tina must have known more than most people that with bipolar, comes the lows as well as the highs and I can imagine that she must have been angry with herself for getting personally involved in my life.

On Friday I did some more unpacking and putting pictures up etc. I couldn't face going outside and walking about in the village because I really didn't want to bump into anyone I knew and have to explain what had happened to me. The intercom buzzed several times while Tina was out but I figured that it must have been Darren and ignored it and sat in the living room in darkness. We went to bed that night and I held Tina in my arms while we looked at the stars and after she finally went to sleep, I thought about seeing my daughter in the morning and went to sleep feeling a bit happier.

Saturday, 12:05pm.

I came out of the church hall into the glaring sunshine but the weather did absolutely nothing to improve my state of mind or the awful feeling of helplessness that had overcome me. I'd spent the last two hours sitting at a desk with my daughter opposite me and the time had just flown by. It felt like I'd only been with her for ten minutes and now I had to wait another two weeks until I saw her again. My phone rang and it was my mum saying that she and Pauline were in the car park of the local swimming pool, just up the road. I got in my car with tears in my eyes and drove the short distance to meet up with them. As I pulled into the car park, I could see my mum's car and pulled up next to it, wiping away the tears so they wouldn't know I was upset. They both gave me a hug and kissed me and then we walked to a Subways for something to eat. I wasn't in the least bit hungry and so just had a coffee and they asked me how my visit had gone. It was really difficult to not start crying and I remember looking down at the table, finding it almost impossible to make eye contact. I must have been mumbling something about how terrible it was to have to walk away from the church hall and can remember just wanting to talk to them in private and not be surrounded by other people eating their food. As soon as they had both finished their sandwiches, I asked if we could go back to my mum's car because I wasn't feeling too good.

Making our way back, I remember starting to panic due to the amount of people everywhere and I couldn't wait to be sat in the car. We eventually arrived at the swimming pool car park but there were still people bustling about all over the place and suddenly I started gasping for breath and had to turn my gaze away, every time somebody walked past. I started to plead with Pauline to get me back to the car and I think that was the first time they noticed how bad I was. Pauline sat in the front and I sat in the back with my mum. I was in a terrible state and remember saying that it felt like I would never see my daughter again and then I put my head on my mum's lap and cried my eyes out. It took about twenty minutes for me to calm down and I eventually asked them if they would like to come and see the flat. They both agreed, so I got in my own car and they started to follow me back to the village. God knows what they must have been saying about me but I'm sure they were both extremely concerned. On the way back, I sent Tina a text to let her know my mum and sister were coming round because I thought it only fair not to surprise her. When we arrived, Pauline asked if I was okay and I told her that I felt a bit better. I introduced them both to Tina and then showed them around the flat and while my mum was talking to her in the kitchen, Pauline and I went out onto the balcony.

"Tina's really nice John"

"I know she is but...."

"But what?"

"I don't love her" (I thought I had but I was wrong)

"Sometimes it can take time to fall in love with someone"

I was feeling so low and when we went back inside, we sat on the sofa and I started to cry again. Tina was saying something to my mum but I didn't know what, I just had this awful feeling that I wasn't going to see the kids again. Eventually, Pauline said that they had better be going and I followed them downstairs to my mum's car. We hugged and as they drove away, I waved and looked at them both for as long as possible before they disappeared from view.

"I'm so sorry Tina," I said when I went back upstairs, "but I've got to go and live with my mum and dad"
"I thought you were going to say that," she replied and went off to the bedroom, shutting the door behind her.
It felt terrible doing that to Tina and right at that moment, I wished I hadn't flirted with her in the hospital and I'm sure she felt exactly the same.
I can't remember how many days passed before I actually left but it must have been within the week. Tina told me that she didn't know anyone in the village and didn't know what she was going to do. I really felt awful and guilty but knew I had to go because as well as for myself, I realised that it would be the best thing for both of us in the long run. It just wasn't fair on her that she was stuck with this thoroughly depressed individual and I couldn't see myself getting any better in the near future.
The wardrobes had only just arrived a few days earlier and I promised I would come back soon and make them up for her.
"I don't really care now," she replied.
I'm sorry Tina, I ruined your life but I really don't know what to say….only that I am so very, very sorry.

CHAPTER 43

February 2009

I arrived at my mum and dad's at about seven in the evening and rang the doorbell. My mum answered and when I went into the living room; my dad was watching the T.V with my nephew Steve. He'd recently split up from his girlfriend and now he too was staying at my parent's house. I suppose they felt it would be a good thing for me if he was there too, as he would be good company. I said hello to them both and then went into the kitchen and sat down at the dining table. My mum came in and made me a cup of tea and then went back into the living room, sensing that I wanted to be on my own. Steve didn't come out for about an hour, probably because my mum had told him to give me some time to myself but when he eventually did, we started to talk and even though I wasn't in the mood, I appreciated him trying to help me. I'll have to skip through the next couple of weeks because all they entail is me crying and sleeping and feeling totally helpless, staring at photos of the children and texting my wife to see if we could get back together again. Steve was out of work at the time and spent most days out somewhere or other, which to be honest I was grateful for because I just didn't feel up to socialising. One day, I was looking through the drawers of a cabinet in the living room; searching for some more photographs and came upon one of me and my wife on our wedding day. I sat down on the sofa and stared at it with tears in my eyes, whispering, "I love you," over and over again.

I sent her a text, asking if I could visit and to my surprise she agreed and so a few days later, I drove back up to Essex hoping that everything could go back how it used to be and it would all be okay again. I set off early and before leaving, sent Tina a text saying that I'd pop in first and start to put the wardrobes together. It was the last thing I wanted to do but promised I would and wanted to see how she was getting on. The atmosphere was really awkward and as I spent most of the time making the wardrobes in the bedroom, she sat in the living room watching T.V. I'd told her that I was going to see my wife and kids and she asked if there was any chance I would get back together with them.

"I don't know," I replied.

"Do you want to get back with your wife?"

"I think so; I want to be with my children"

"I miss my son too," she said.

As soon as I pulled up outside my old house, something just didn't feel right; it didn't seem like home any more. My wife answered the door and then my daughter rushed past her and gave me a great big hug. I found it so difficult to not just burst out crying and it was brilliant to be with her again. Both my boys were there and I remember feeling ashamed that I'd been sectioned but they were both absolutely fine with me. It must sound that I am not as close to my sons as I am to my daughter and from the point of view that I don't see them as much, then that is true but I love them all equally as much and am very proud of them.

SECTION 3: LOW

We just never went into all that hugging and "I love you son" stuff because I stupidly thought it to be not very manly. It's such a ridiculous way to be and all my own fault but I really do love you boys. For some reason, when my daughter was born, I changed and was able to show my feeling so much more. Whereas I would give her a hug, I would pat the boys on the shoulder but would do it in a sort of jokey way. They have got the same sense of humour as me and I'm sure they both know how I feel about them. I remember playing draughts with my daughter and feeling so safe in her company. That sounds like a really odd thing to say but she'll never know how much she helped me get through all of this. I suppose it was her naivety, not understanding what had happened and me not having to explain it all to her. That evening after she'd gone to bed, I stood in the kitchen talking to my wife, asking her if I could come back home again. I was totally confused and contradicting myself, knowing this didn't feel like my home any more and yet wanting to come back at the same time.

"Too much has happened John," she replied, "It could never be the same again"

Deep down I knew she was right and if I'm totally honest, I didn't really want to get back with her but wanted to be with the kids and I'm sure she felt the same about me. I still loved my wife, I just didn't know it for a while and I'm sure I always will. After being together for over twenty years, you really get to know someone inside out and we had some wonderful times together. I suppose our main problem was money worries as it is with most couples and after years of it, the strain became too much. We both didn't know it at the time but I had and always will have bipolar disorder and just didn't seem to take our financial situation that seriously. It would always be her who had to deal with any problems and I'm sorry if it seemed like I didn't care. She is a 100% decent person and never asked for anything and is probably the hardest worker I have ever met; I'm just not as strong as her. I said that I love my wife and I do but not how I used to, we are now good friends and I hope we will be for ever. She said that I could stay the night, on the sofa-bed downstairs and my daughter gave me one of her Paddington Bears to cuddle which I did, feeling the love and affection she had given it. I fell asleep squeezing Paddington and crying my eyes out (yet again)

The next morning, I gave the kids a hug and said goodbye to them. My daughter was going to school and my wife worked there also, as a teaching assistant. My two boys were still at college and both left together in my eldest son's car. I'd asked my wife if I could get some stuff out of the loft to take back to my mum and dad's and she agreed, telling me to make sure I shut the front door behind me when I left. My plan was to load the car up and then drive over to Tina's and carry on putting the wardrobes together. After I'd got what I wanted out of the loft, I made myself a cup of tea and then went on the computer in the spare room downstairs. I was going to see if I had any emails because I hadn't checked them since before I was sectioned but noticed that my wife hadn't signed out after checking hers. I looked at her sent messages and saw one sent to her mother a few days earlier. It mentioned all these things about how scared my wife had been when I tried to visit her a couple of weeks before I'd been put in the hospital and how I'd been recently asking her if we could get back together. She wrote that would never happen now and the thought that I would never be back in the family home again with the kids, made me fall apart. I sat on the end of the sofa-bed which I still hadn't put back up and started shaking uncontrollably. Tears were streaming down my face and I kept repeating to myself over and over again, "What am I going to do?"

I stared up into the corner of the room and can't really describe the pain I felt inside. I was a total wreck and sent my wife a text, asking if I could stay until she came home that afternoon with my daughter. I didn't get any reply but a short while later; she pulled up on the drive and came in. I was still on the sofa-bed weeping and she asked me what was wrong. Between bouts of sobbing, I managed to say that I'd read her email to her mum and now knew that I could never come back.

"I know you don't want to come back because of me John but because of the children. My feelings have changed towards you too and I know we can't go back to how it used to be"

"Can I at least stay until the kids get home, so I can say goodbye?"

"You said goodbye this morning. I know it seems like I'm being really hard on you but I don't want them to see you like this and think that it's best if you go now"

I knew she was right and couldn't think of anything to say in response.

"You can visit again John," she said, "lets just do this slowly and we can speak on the phone in the mean time"

BIPOLAR.....ME?

Getting up, I gave her a kiss on the cheek and apologised for all that had happened.
"I've got to get back to work," she said, "Don't forget to shut the door behind you"
"That's okay, I'll leave at the same time as you. I've loaded up the car already"
She kissed me on the cheek and said she'd ring me later.
Driving back to Tina's, I sent her a text to let her know I'd be with her shortly but really wasn't in the mood to set foot in the flat. Once I got there, she asked me how I was but I could see she wasn't too good herself. I said I was sorry over and over again and after putting a couple of drawers together, I told her that I had to go. The crisis team had arranged for me to see a psychiatrist every two weeks, a short distance from the hospital and I was due to see him on the coming Friday. It was totally inconvenient because I was now living with my parents and it meant a round trip of two hundred and seventy miles, just for a half hour meeting but I figured that I could get to see the kids while in the area and told Tina I would come back and finish the wardrobes at the same time. On my way back to my parent's house, I was driving on the M3 heading for Hampshire and was doing a top speed of fifty mph. I was feeling so low and didn't want to have to concentrate too much on driving and so figured it would be best to stay in the slow lane. It was a lovely sunny day without a cloud in the sky but my mind was full of dark and depressing thoughts and it would have actually been better if the weather was damp and grey. I absolutely love music and tried to lift my spirits by putting on a load of my favourite songs but nothing worked. Tracks which had once been so

important to me meant nothing and I had to switch the stereo off. On several occasions, I was so close to turning the steering wheel quickly to the left and crashing down an embankment because I just wanted the pain to go away. When I eventually arrived back at my mum and dad's, they asked me how everything went but I didn't want to talk and shut myself in my bedroom with the curtains drawn. The following day, I had my car repossessed and it was actually a relief. It meant now that I didn't have to worry about the repayments, not that I was really that bothered anyway. The way I was feeling, they could have locked me up and I wouldn't have cared less.

Friday.
I asked my dad if I could borrow his car because I had to see the psychiatrist and rang my wife to check if it would be okay if I came round to visit afterwards. A female member of the crisis team I knew from the hospital was waiting with the psychiatrist when I turned up. From being this person brimming with confidence the last time I had seen her, I was now this empty shell, completely withdrawn. The doctor had never seen me any differently and she explained to him, how much I had changed. I remember saying sorry to her for all the problems I had caused the crisis team and she explained that she'd found me to be totally intimidating. I was really surprised by this and said I wasn't like that normally. The doctor asked me if I had seen my wife and how the relationship was going and for some reason, I lied and said there was a good chance we were going to get back together.
"Are you still taking your medication John?" he asked.
"Yes," I lied.

BIPOLAR…..ME?

It seems completely crazy to me now but I still wasn't taking the meds and I have no idea why. Finally, he said that he'd see me in a couple of weeks' time and then I drive over to my wife's house. Both the boys were out with their mates but my daughter was there and it was so great to see her again. While she was taking a bath, I started talking to my wife and got upset again.

"Are you taking the tablets?" she asked.

"No," I sobbed.

"You've got to John, it will help you to cope with the situation and stop you from crying all of the time"

"I don't need any tablets"

"Yes you do and if you don't start taking them straight away, I'll phone the hospital and tell them"

"Why? Why can't you just let me get through this my own way?"

"Because you need them to get back on track. I hated it, you having to see our little girl at that place every other Saturday but didn't know how you were going to behave mentally and had to think of her. If you don't start taking the tablets, then I've got no choice but to stop you seeing her again!"

I suddenly realised and appreciated the position she was in. All along I thought she was just being vindictive by making me see our daughter under supervision but now understood that she was worried for her safety. I don't mean she thought I was going to hurt her, of course I wasn't and my wife knew that but because of my bipolar, I was unpredictable and she was concerned that I might not look after her properly.

"I will start taking them, I promise," and this time I meant it.

SECTION 3: LOW

I reached into my pocket, pulled out a box of meds (Sodium Valproate) and got a glass of water before taking one.

"Why do you carry them around with you, if you're not taking them?" she asked.

"So when the doctor asks me if I'm still on them, I can get them out and show them to him but you have my word; I will definitely carry on taking them every day from now on"

CHAPTER 44

March 2009

I was out of work for two reasons. The first one because there wasn't that much available but the overriding reason was, I just wasn't able to work. My self confidence had plummeted to zero and I struggled to go for a walk, let alone get a job. Physically, there was nothing wrong with me and if someone knew I wasn't working, they would have probably thought I was just another person sponging off the state and would rather lay about the house all day doing nothing. I must admit if I had been in their position, I would have thought exactly the same but until you go through a state of total and absolute depression, nobody else can fully understand how it feels (fucking horrible! That's the answer!)

I would wake up every morning and the thought of getting through another day, would send me into an even lower mood. Every part of my body ached and it felt as if I were walking along under water, the simplest tasks becoming a struggle. I've always been someone who's found some sort of pride in not getting stressed about things and over the years, I have been in some very stressful situations but not let them get to me. There was this guy at a place I used to work at and he would try everything possible to stress me out but he was wasting his time, I was immune. It's only now in hindsight, that I can see a certain amount of stress is probably a good thing from time to time. People have told me that I'm very laid back (when I'm level) which is all very well but at some time, you have to snap and that has happened to me on a couple of occasions but it is extremely rare. The crisis team had given me the number of an organisation called MIND who give support and advice to people suffering from mental health issues. At first I wasn't interested but in the end, I gave them a ring and they suggested that I contact Shaw Trust (a charity which supports disabled and disadvantaged people to prepare for work and help find them jobs) They arranged for me to go for an interview with one of their development officers, which was basically someone trying to find you a suitable job. I remember sitting in front of this bloke and not being able to look at him in the eye because I was so low and lacking in confidence. He was really patient with me and understood that it would take time, explaining that when I was eventually ready to go back to work, it would give me some sort of self worth and that in turn, would lift my spirits and increase my confidence. Of course I knew that already but it was nice to have someone understand how I felt. I was due to see him again the following week.

My mum and dad would go to the supermarket every day to get a newspaper and a few bits and would always ask me if I wanted to come. Most of the time I would say no and just sit at home reading books (I felt that helped me because I didn't need to speak to anybody) but on the odd occasions I did go with them, I would always wait in the car while they went shopping. I couldn't face being amongst crowds of people and had become totally withdrawn. Steve was out of work also at this point and it did help to some degree, him being around. I hadn't had a beer for about seven weeks (which was a miracle for me) and I remember saying to Steve one day, "Do you fancy a drink?"

"We're both skint!" he replied.

We walked down to the supermarket and I stole a case of twenty four beers and then we drank them in the park. I'd never shoplifted before (apart from sweets when I was a kid) but when you haven't got any money and are really not able to work, it's amazing how quickly your attitude changes. With the little money we did have (the majority of mine was spent on cigarettes) we'd go down the pub and buy one beer each and keep topping them up with cans we had stashed outside. We would sit in the beer garden, so not to arouse the suspicion of the landlord and every now and then, go in and play a game of pool. Steve is a good player but I couldn't believe how much my game had deteriorated. I was missing the easiest of shots and didn't know what was wrong with me. Over the course of the next few weeks, I was stealing cases of beer on a regular basis but the drinking wasn't helping my depression in the slightest. Naively, I thought it would lift my spirits but deep down I knew that alcohol heightens whatever mood you happen to be in, either high or low. The thought of getting caught shoplifting, didn't bother me in the slightest; I just didn't care.

April 2009

Lucy rang me and asked how I was getting on. I didn't want her to know how low I was really feeling because she sounded quite cheerful and I didn't want her to worry about me.

SECTION 3: LOW

"Yeh, I'm doing good Luce," I lied, "how are you?"
"I've stopped smoking!"
"I don't believe it, you of all people!"
"I know, Stewart has been encouraging me to quit and I've finally done it. I've put on a load of weight though"
"That's only natural, how is Stewart?"
"He's fine and says hello"
"That's good" (I was finding it really difficult to sound happy and couldn't wait to get off the phone) "I've got to go now Luce," I said, "I'll speak to you soon. Look after yourself"
That was the last time I ever spoke to Lucy. She probably thought I didn't want to talk to her but that wasn't entirely true. I didn't want to talk to anyone because I wasn't fun to be around and only hope she is still doing well and is still with Stewart. You never knew it Lucy but you were my absolute hero and still are, I respect you so much.
A couple of days later, Zee rang me.
"All right son, how yer doing?" he bellowed.
I was feeling exactly the same and so after telling him I was okay, I quickly asked what he had been up to. It turned out that he was living with his parents also and was still seeing the crisis team and a psychiatrist on a regular basis. I told him that I'd talk to him soon and I wasn't wrong because he kept on ringing me almost every day from then on. It's not that I didn't like Zee (I do, very much) but being in contact with the guys from the hospital wasn't making me feel any better and I just wanted to forget about the whole experience. Every other week, I would drive up to Essex to see my psychiatrist and then go and see the kids. It was clear to me by now that my wife didn't want our

relationship to return to us living together again and when the doctor asked me about this subject, I told him the truth. I explained to him that the real reason I wanted to get back together with her was because I wanted to be with the kids and he said that would be a big mistake. I knew he was right but was lying to myself, hoping it would all be okay again as if nothing had happened. When he asked me if I was still taking the tablets, I replied that I was but they weren't helping my depression. He explained they were designed to stop me having big highs or lows but they were clearly not working on the low department. I asked if he could prescribe me some anti-depressants and he was hesitant at first, concerned that they might return me to a high state again but in the end agreed, telling me to call him immediately if I showed any signs of abnormal euphoria. Each time I drove back to Hampshire, the urge to crash the car became greater and greater. Even though I was seeing the kids more often, it made it all the harder every time I said goodbye. Steve bought a dongle for my laptop and I found Tina on Facebook. When I had left the flat for good, I deleted her number on my mobile, thinking it best not to get in touch with her again. I asked how she was getting on and she explained that she'd gone back to her husband and had come to an agreement with the landlord, selling the furniture to him so he could rent the place out as furnished. Once again, I said how sorry I was the way things had turned out and she replied that it was okay and for me to take care. After I typed back that she take care too, I deleted her as a friend and was relieved that she'd managed to sort things out with the landlord. I hope you are doing well Tina and everything is okay.

CHAPTER 45

May 2009, Saturday night

Steve had gone out and I was sitting in the kitchen, watching television. Over the course of the next couple of hours I drank ten cans of Stella, stuck my head round the living room door, said goodnight to my mum and dad and went upstairs to my bedroom. Lying in bed in the darkness, I was crying my eyes out and was the lowest I'd ever felt. It just seemed like the pain wouldn't go away and so I got up, switched the light on, took all of my Sodium Valproate tablets and all of my anti-depressants and then went back to bed. I remember lying there; thinking that I could feel my toes wiggle and my arms move and that it might be the last time I had those sensations. Looking back now, I really don't know what I wanted to happen. I don't believe in life after death and so knew that if I did die, then that was it, there would be nothing ever again. People always say to someone who has attempted suicide and have children, "But what about your kids, how can you do that to them?"

The truth is, when you are that low, nothing makes sense any more and you're clearly not in a right frame of mind. I don't think I really wanted to die, it was more a cry for help and I hoped that if I did wake up again, everything would be better. My dad found me unconscious on the bathroom floor and managed to revive me and then the next thing I remember was being back in my bed with two paramedics standing above me, asking lots of questions and giving me an injection. My dad was at the foot of the bed; crying and I shut my eyes.

The two paramedics were helping me down the stairs and I must have shut my eyes again because I was then lying in the back of an ambulance with my mum sitting next to me. Pauline might have been there too, I can't recall. I shut my eyes and the next thing I remember was sitting behind a curtain in a hospital ward and mum, dad, Pauline and her husband Dave were stood all around me. I closed my eyes again and the next time I opened them it was daylight and my sister Ellie was sitting on the end of the hospital bed, gently stroking my hand with a drip attached to it. She had tears in her eyes and I remember thinking, "Oh shit, what the fuck have I done?!"

It's difficult to explain how I was feeling when I woke up. It was nice to see Ellie and a big part of me was extremely relieved that I was alive and okay but there was also a part that wished I was dead. I'd thought the night before that if I did survive, then everything would be okay again but I still felt totally miserable and the pain was still there. Ellie didn't ask me why I had done it; she just smiled and continued to stroke my hand.

"Can you take me home?" I asked her.

She nodded and said, "I'll see what the nurse says," and then went off to find someone.

While she was gone, I pulled the drip out of my hand and sat up on the edge of the bed, feeling a bit dizzy. When Ellie came back, she said that the doctor wanted to see me first and would be round in about an hour. I started to get dressed and Ellie went to get a couple of coffees.

SECTION 3: LOW

The doctor finally showed up and said that I had been very lucky because I'd apparently been sick at home before passing out and had got rid of most of the tablets before they had a chance to absorb into my bloodstream. I remember telling him that I was very sorry and he told me that I could go and not to ever attempt anything like that again. On the journey back home, I stared out of the passenger window and didn't say a word to Ellie. My mum and dad were waiting in the kitchen when we got back and I mumbled, "Sorry," to them and then went to bed and slept for the next six hours.

Sunday evening.
It was only when I woke up at about eight that night, that I thought to myself, "What a stupid thing to do, I'm so fucking stupid!"
I was so cross with myself and felt what I was going through was nothing compared to some people and I know it sounds strange but I think that experience was a kick up the arse for me. It actually made me appreciate life again and I'm not saying from that very moment, everything was good again but over the course of the next few months, my mood did start to slowly lift. A few days after the overdose, I got a call from Dominique. She was back at home, living with her parents and didn't sound like the same person I remembered from the hospital ward. I told her what I had done and she started to cry, saying that she felt suicidal too.
"Please don't do it," I said, "Please, please don't do it. Things will get better"
"Have they for you?" she sobbed.

"No, not really….not yet anyway but I just know that it will improve"
"I can't see things ever improving"
"They will, they've got to. I'm a lot like you and we're both suffering from the same thing. You love life too much and those feelings will come back"
"I fucking hate life!"
"At the moment you do, so do I but please try to get through it!"
"I'll try," she whispered.
"Do you promise?"
"Yes"
"Can I ring you next week?" I asked.
"Yes, I want you to"
"I'll speak to you soon Dominique, please take care"
"Bye John"
It's funny but although I hadn't wanted to talk to Lucy and Zee, I felt so much better after that call with Dominique. She was obviously as depressed as I was and I suppose it was selfish of me to feel slightly better but I felt we were very much alike and I could relate to her. Unlike Lucy who had been through absolute hell in her life and I could never even begin to imagine what that must have been like, Dominique and I had both experienced massive highs while suffering from bipolar and were now on the come down. We'd both had pretty privileged lives growing up and when it got to the stage where we could do whatever we pleased (she in her early twenties and me when I'd turned forty and lived on my own for the first time in years) we both went off the rails. The following Friday, I saw my psychiatrist again and he'd obviously been informed about the overdose. By this stage, I was really beginning to not only accept help

but actually want it too. He told me that if I hadn't spewed up that night, then there was a very good chance I could have gone into a coma and totally screwed up my insides (not his actual words but you get my drift)

I told him that I was really sorry and would never ever do it again. It seemed to be so impractical to have to drive such a distance to see him each time and I asked if I could be transferred to another doctor, closer to my parent's house. He appeared to be slightly miffed by this at first but I explained that I'd like to see someone on a weekly basis and the cost in fuel was too much for me. I think he realised what I was going on about and said he'd contact my G.P in Hampshire and ask him to refer me to a local psychiatrist. I thanked him for all his help and once again, promised to never take an overdose again. The following week, I called Dominique to see how she was getting on.

"I just mope about the house all day, I don't feel any better," she answered.

"Have you tried reading any books?" I asked.

"I fucking hate reading!"

"Try it, I find it helps me. It takes your mind off things and it's just you and the book and your imagination"

She said that she'd give it a go and would call me in a couple of days.

CHAPTER 46

June 2009

My brother-in-law Dave is the chef at a registered charity organisation which cares and houses people with learning difficulties. They are a non-profit organisation and are always desperate for volunteers. He suggested that I go and look at the place and if I liked it, then I could possibly apply as a volunteer myself. Dave said that the atmosphere of the place would be really good for me and would also help to get my confidence back again. I must admit that the thought of going to this alien place and not knowing anyone apart from Dave, terrified me but I was determined to do it. I knew I had to force myself if I ever hoped to get any better and would have by far wanted to be in a work environment where I at least knew one person, opposed to everybody being a total stranger. So one day the following week, I borrowed my dad's car and drove to Dave's place of work. Steve came with me as I didn't know where it was and waited in the car, while I went in search of my brother-in-law. I'd turned off a country lane and there was this long sweeping drive lined with trees and flowers, which led to the courtyard of this beautiful old building. There were lots of people walking around and it was clear to me that some of them had learning difficulties and I asked one of them where the kitchen was. He was really friendly and asked me my name, then told me his and took me to see Dave, who seemed really pleased to see me and introduced me to some of the guys helping him in the kitchen. After we spoke for a while, he telephoned one of the day service managers to let him know I had arrived and when he came into the kitchen, he shook my hand and said his name was Peter. He seemed such a nice and friendly man and asked me if I was ready for a tour of the place. I was still very insecure and I suppose it came across as me being shy but it didn't seem to bother him and he showed me all around these amazing rooms. There was the pottery department, full of people working away and they all said hello to me in such a pleasant and genuine way. The room was full of shelves and on top of them were all different kinds of pottery and figures, created by the service users; I was well impressed. Peter showed me the gardens which were beautiful and not only had a huge array of flowers but also many different kinds of vegetables, which Dave used every day for his dishes. After that, he took me into the art class and I remember this girl shouting out, "Hello, whoever you are!"

That was the first time I'd laughed in ages and I could feel this complete sense of kindness, emanating from everyone. I was struck by the fact that everyone seemed so happy and the whole place had a lovely feel about it.

Peter then took me into the woodwork room and all of the guys in there said hello and showed me all the tools and machinery. When he'd finished giving me the tour, Peter got me some forms to fill in and asked me some questions about hobbies and interests etc.

"So John, do you think you'd like to work here as a volunteer?" he asked.

"Yes, I really like what I've seen and everyone seems so friendly"

"Is there anything in particular that you feel you'd like to do?"

"Well….Dave said that he could always do with some more help in the kitchen, so perhaps I could start off by doing that"

The truth was that I still didn't feel comfortable in the presence of strangers and felt that by working with Dave, I could slowly get to know everybody. Peter said that they would have to do a CRB check on me (Criminal Records Bureau) which is standard procedure for anyone wishing to work with vulnerable people and it could take up to three months to get a reply back. We shook hands and before leaving, I popped into the kitchen to see Dave again.

"How did it go?" he asked.

"Yeh, really good. It could take three months to get my CRB though"

"So you'd like to become a volunteer?"

"Yes, definitely!"

"That's great John, I'm really pleased and don't forget that it could eventually lead to a paid position here" (He's such a nice bloke!)

"That would be handy!"

"How d'ya get on?" asked Steve when I got back in the car.

"Yeh, I really liked it but I've got to wait for a CRB check to be done"

"You'll have no trouble there; it just takes a bit of time to come through"

The next couple of months really dragged by, waiting to get the CRB check and being totally skint was

SECTION 3: LOW

starting to get me down but I promised myself not to shoplift again. I rang Dominique to see how she was getting on and she sounded a lot more cheerful but definitely not how I remembered her in the hospital (a good thing I suppose) I'd told Steve about her dad being in the construction industry and perhaps he'd be able to get a job for us both. When I asked her if she thought it was possible, the tone in her voice changed immediately. She was still friendly but I could tell she felt the only reason I rang her was to see if I could get a job. It was partly true but my main concern was her well being and straight away, I wished I'd never said anything.

"I don't know John," she replied, "I don't really like to ask him"

"That's okay mate," I said, "It was just a thought"

Looking back now, it wouldn't have worked anyway and I obviously wasn't thinking straight. I lived in Hampshire now and her dad's business was in Essex; how would I have got there each day? After talking to her for about ten more minutes, we said goodbye and I hung up. I've never spoken to Dominique since.

Of course, when we were admitted into the hospital, we were both at the peak of a bipolar high and it's such an irrational state to be in but it was a laugh and we had some real good times. I miss you mate and hope all is well. I was still seeing the guy at Shaw Trust on a regular basis and he kept saying that my confidence would slowly return and by getting a job, that would speed up the process considerably. He suggested several vacancies, working in hotel kitchens etc but Dave had told me that the man running the woodwork dept at the organisation he worked at, was considering retirement in the not too distant future and

I was starting to pin my hopes on filling that position. I mentioned this to the Shaw Trust guy and told him that I had already applied to be a volunteer and he seemed to be very enthusiastic about the whole thing. My G.P phoned a few days later and asked if I would go and see him that afternoon. When I got there, he said that he'd received a phone call from my psychiatrist in Essex, explaining that I wished to be transferred to a doctor much closer to where I now lived. He agreed that it made much more sense and then told me that he'd arranged for me to see a psychiatrist at a clinic just up the road.

"Great!" I replied.

"There's just one thing," he said.

"What's that?"

"It's the same doctor you took a particular disliking to, when he and a colleague came to see you at your sister's house, along with the social worker"

"Oh"

"Do you have a problem with that?"

In my mind, I visualised myself at Pauline and Dave's house the night I was sectioned and remembered the hatred I felt towards the psychiatrist. At the time, he seemed to be so arrogant to me but those feelings had completely vanished and I now felt embarrassment instead of anger. I now understood that they were there to help me and I relayed this to my G.P.

"Are you sure it won't be problematic and cause you unwanted distress?" he asked.

Somehow, I knew it would be the best thing for me to see the psychiatrist again.

"Yes, I'm sure," I answered.

"Good, then I'll get in touch with him and arrange for you to see him as soon as possible"

SECTION 3: LOW

Things had really started to improve with my wife. I'd finally accepted that I was never going back to the house and she could sense that. I was still finding it extremely difficult, saying goodbye to my daughter each time I visited (by now, both my boys had left college and were working and not at home most of the time I visited) but at least now when I drove back to Hampshire, I didn't have the urge to crash the car. As I mentioned earlier, the overdose incident had made me see the light if you like and the thought of never seeing the kids again, was unbearable. Each time I drove back to my parent's, I couldn't wait to see them again and that helped to lift my spirits. A letter came for me in the post several days later; informing me I had an appointment to see the psychiatrist the following week. I'd told Pauline it was the same doctor who'd had me sectioned and she explained that he was a really nice man and had comforted her after the police had taken me away. She told me not to worry and just be myself but above all, tell him the truth. I promised I would and could finally see the logic of being completely honest with a person who was qualified to help me. And so the next week, I went to see him but found it hard to look him in the eye because I was feeling so ashamed at how I'd behaved. Pauline was right, he was a nice man and told me not to feel awkward and that it was a positive thing that I felt the way I did.

"It shows you are getting better John because you now realise those thoughts were irrational and not how you really feel," he explained.

He put me completely at ease and without even realising it, I was now giving him full eye contact and we were having long conversations. At the end of my appointment, I shook his hand and apologised for my behaviour that evening. He patted me on the arm and in a light-hearted fashion said, "You were a bit anti me, to say the least"

"I'm so sorry," I replied sheepishly.

"Don't worry John; it's just good to see you back on track. Take care and I'll see you in a couple of weeks"

Driving home, I was feeling so much better. It made complete sense that I see this man; he was there when I was sectioned and by listening to what he had to say regarding my mental state at the time, could only help me understand my condition and deal with it. The next time I visited my wife, I asked her if there was any chance my daughter could come and stay one weekend at my mum and dad's house. To my total surprise, she agreed and we arranged to meet at Fleet services on the M3, which is roughly the halfway point between where we both live. I now realise how difficult it must have been for my wife to make that decision because her prime concern was the safety of our daughter and she obviously felt that because I was taking my medication and seeing the doctor on a regular basis, I wasn't going to do anything silly like driving mad or something along those lines. Not that I ever would have but it was nice to know she felt comfortable enough to trust me. The next time I saw the psychiatrist, I told him the news and he seemed genuinely pleased for me.

"Things do seem to be starting to change around for you John," he said.

It seemed to take an eternity but the Friday afternoon came when I was to meet my wife and daughter at Fleet. I was so excited as I made my way there and as

SECTION 3: LOW

I pulled up in the car park, I could see my daughter waving at me from the back seat of my wife's car. She had a big beaming smile on her face and words could never do justice how that made me feel inside. She gave me a great big hug and said she was looking forward to seeing nanny and pops. I loaded her stuff into the boot of my dad's car and after kissing my wife goodbye and promising to text her when we got home, we set off. On the journey back, my daughter wouldn't stop talking and it was joy to my ears. I loved her innocence and the fact that she seemed totally oblivious to everything that had gone on. The journey from Fleet takes a little over one hour and when we were driving down this country lane, she said, "I can remember seeing a fox here a long time ago. It was night time then and the lights from your car, made his eyes glow in the dark"

We've drove down that road loads of times since and each time we reach that point, she says the same thing. My mum and dad loved seeing her again and to have her in my company without being watched over in a hall somewhere or even with her mum, made me feel so happy. Don't get me wrong, I've nothing against my wife but it just felt so good to be with my daughter and we could spend some time to ourselves. The weather was lovely that weekend and we went crabbing at a place called Mudeford, about six miles away from my parent's house. While everyone else around us seemed to be pulling up loads of crabs, we only caught one but that didn't seem to bother her and she called him "Pinchy"

She's such a great kid and never asks for anything (just as well, I'm skint. Ha ha!) and takes such pleasure in enjoying the simple things in life. She loves nature and looking under rocks and stones, searching for weird and wonderful insects and it's an absolute joy being in her company.

The weekend went all too quickly and after dropping her off back to her mum at Fleet, I drove home and kept turning round to look at the empty seat she had been sitting in. I started to become tearful, wishing she was still in my company but found comfort in the fact that she could come and stay again soon. The problem was that I had too much time on my hands and I needed something to take my mind off all the negative thoughts. It seemed to be taking for ever, waiting for the CRB to come through and most of my days were filled with thinking about my kids and how much I missed them.

CHAPTER 47

September 2009

At last the CRB finally arrived and gave the all clear for me to start as a volunteer at Dave's place. I phoned the organisation to let them know and they said that they'd just received it too and when would I like to start.
"As soon as possible!" I replied.
They asked me how many days a week I would like to work and I suggested Mondays, Tuesdays and Thursdays. Although I couldn't wait to start just to take my mind off things, I was still anxious about working with strangers and felt that three days a week would be enough for the moment. Dave picked me up the following Monday morning and we got there before anyone else had arrived, apart from a service users who lived in the flats upstairs but none of the others had come down yet. Being the chef, Dave always likes to get there early and start prepping the food and so I helped him by chopping up some vegetables. After about twenty minutes, a service user called Adam walked into the kitchen and said good morning to Dave.
"Morning Adam," he replied, "this is my brother-in-law John and he's starting as a volunteer in the kitchen"
I didn't know it at the time but Adam had a pub kitchen job in a town about three miles down the road on Tuesdays and Wednesdays but helped Dave in his

kitchen for the rest of the week. He smiled at me and said good morning and then went off somewhere. Next, in walked a girl with a walking stick and she gave me a great big smile and said good morning. I found myself being immediately relaxed and happy to be in the company of these people. By 9am, more and more service users started to arrive and quite a few of them came into the kitchen to say hello to Dave. He introduced all of them to me but I found it really difficult trying to remember their names, as there were so many of them. I spent all of that first day in the kitchen, occasionally going into the courtyard for a cigarette and can remember at lunchtime as we served up, all of the staff coming into the kitchen to help serve up the food to the guys and them all saying hello to me. Thinking back now, I really can't remember any of them and recently asked the girl in the art department how I seemed to her on that day. She said I appeared extremely shy and just kept my head down, hardly making eye contact with anyone. Because I'd been out of work for so long, it seemed like such a long day and by the end of it I was knackered and couldn't wait to get home. It sounds really silly now but I'd become so withdrawn and hadn't spoken to so many people for so long, I think it wore me out.

It was at about this time that my dad started to become ill. He would go to the toilet and obviously be in some discomfort as we could hear him groaning with pain. He'd been going to see his G.P for a couple of years previous to this and the doctor couldn't find anything wrong but now, the pain was clearly starting to escalate. Every time I came home from work of an evening, it became so hard listening to him in agony.

SECTION 3: LOW

My sister booked another appointment at the surgery and they did some tests and after a couple of days when they came back, it still showed there was nothing wrong. As each day passed and I went to work as a volunteer, my confidence started to slowly get better but I was nowhere near my old self. It was a strange time for me; I was feeling better in myself and yet this sensation was counterbalanced by my dad's illness and that obviously slowed down the improvement in my well being. That may come across as me being selfish but I really don't mean it to be, it's just the way I was feeling and it wasn't until much later that I realised it. Recalling it now, it's like my feelings were on some sort of roller coaster: one day happy and feeling quite confident and the next, totally miserable and worried about my dad. I will always be extremely grateful to Dave for suggesting I become a volunteer (he knew I would fit in well and get along with the guys) but my confidence didn't really improve until I started to help out in the woodwork department. When I worked in the kitchen, I didn't get to see many of the service users during the course of the day but when I went into woodwork, I got to work alongside the guys and help them make things. I'm bleedin' useless with food (apart from scoffing it!) but love making things and found the guys in woodwork to be like minded.

Every Halloween is celebrated at work with the guys dressing up in scary costumes and getting their faces painted by the art department. Foolishly, I allowed one of the service users to paint my face. Being bald, I thought it would be a good idea to have my head painted like a skull but she made a right pig's ear of it. My face looked like a bomb had hit it but the great thing about that place is you just don't care and I even drove home with the debacle still over me boat race. It was worth it just to see my dad smile but he had become so much worse.

November 2009

It was a Monday morning and I was due to go into work with Dave as usual but my dad was in a terrible state and so I rang him to say I couldn't make it. The doctor had done some more tests a few days earlier and wanted to see him again, so I drove my mum and dad to the surgery and sat in the waiting room while my mum went in with him. They were gone for ages but eventually, my mum poked her head round the door leading to the doctor's rooms and whispered for me to come in. When I shut the door behind me, I could see my mum was upset and asked her what was wrong.
"He's got cancer all over and there's nothing they can do," she replied.
We went into this room and my dad was standing up, holding himself against a desk top, crying his eyes out. It was absolutely awful and the doctor tried comforting him but it was no use. He explained to me and my mum that he'd rang Bournemouth Hospital and they were expecting us straight away and rather than wait for an ambulance, it would be quicker if we drove there ourselves. My dad was in a really bad way and the doctor suggested that it would be better if we go out the back way, so he didn't have to go through the waiting room and be seen by all the other patients. He opened the door for us and me and mum had to hold dad either side as he was near to collapsing, then

led us along a corridor which came to a door opening onto the car park at the back of the building. Mum got in the back of the car with dad and he put his head on her lap and I drove us to the hospital as quickly as I could without trying to cause him too much discomfort. When we arrived, I pulled up right outside the main entrance and told my mum I'd park up while they went inside and after getting out the car, I smoked about five fags, one after the other. We'd all known something wasn't right with dad but because the tests had kept coming back as okay, we had assumed that it couldn't have been anything too serious. To me, it all seemed surreal. He woke up at home that morning, in his own bed and now he was in hospital and wasn't coming out ever again.

My sister Jane was due to arrive in England from Sydney at the beginning of December, with her two daughters and her husband Andy. They were all going back in the New Year but because of my dad's condition, Jane decided to take an earlier flight so she could see him and give my mum some support. I can always remember the first time she saw him in the hospital. He'd already been in there a couple of weeks and had deteriorated rapidly and when we arrived in his room, he was in the bathroom. We waited for him for about five minutes and when he came through the door, Jane couldn't help crying but hid it from him as best she could. My dad wasn't a tall man but he seemed to have shrunk and looked about twenty years older, unsteady on his feet and appearing to look confused. It was great to see him smile when he saw Jane and after a while, he actually seemed to improve slightly. Once he was admitted into hospital, dad accepted he was going to die and from that moment on, remained quite cheerful and talkative. It's really strange but during the whole time of my dad's illness, I felt emotionless about the whole thing and it's only as I'm writing this bit now (3 years later) that I'm feeling upset. It's not that I didn't care about him, of course I did but I just felt nothing inside, like I was a blank book. I think it's because I'd been through all these different extremes of emotion and now on medication, was somehow immune to any feelings, either good or bad. My brother Davey would often come down from Essex to visit dad and so it was good he got to see all five of his kids at the same time. One evening, me and Steve went to visit him with my mum and when she went to get a coffee, he motioned me over to the bed and said in almost a whisper "You look after her or I'll come back and haunt you"

In early December, my dad was moved into a hospice and I'm sure everyone who's had a family member or friend go into one will tell you, the staff are absolutely terrific. Me and Jane went to Heathrow a couple of days later to pick up her daughter's and it was lovely to see them again. Andy arrived the following week and my dad died a couple of days later, on 19th December 2009. A year earlier, I was in a nut house and remember thinking that things could only improve by next Christmas. It just goes to show how wrong you can be.

SECTION 4: GETTING BETTER

CHAPTER 48

January 2010

It hadn't been the happiest Christmas I can remember and now Jane and Andy and the girls had gone back home to Australia, everything was returning to normal (or as normal as it could be)
My dad had been the youngest of nine brothers, the youngest of his generation and was the last to go. Now that title goes to me because I'm the youngest of the next generation and that's quite something because there's fucking hundreds of us! I was still seeing the psychiatrist once every couple of months and he was pleased with the way I seemed to be improving. He told me he was sorry to hear about my dad and asked if I needed to up the dosage on my anti-depressants but I told him I was okay. When I was working in the woodwork department the following day, I asked the instructor if it was true that he was retiring soon.
"I've got a farmhouse in France and I'm doing it up," he said.
(I already knew this via Dave but played dumb)
"Are you planning to live there then?" I asked.
"Yes. For the last six months, I've been driving there after work on a Friday afternoon, working on the place and getting back here Sunday evenings"
"That must be knackering"
"It is, that's why I'm going to cut down to only working here two days a week so I can spend more time on the farmhouse"

SECTION 4: GETTING BETTER

"When do you reckon it will be finished?"
"The plan is to be moved in by the beginning of August"
On the way home that night, I mentioned it to Dave and he said that hopefully it was possible I could start getting paid on the days the woodwork guy was in France. He said he'd speak to our manager and see what he thought.

February 2010

My mum asked if I'd like to go to Portugal in ten days time, for two weeks and I said yes. I hadn't been there for years and absolutely love the place. My uncle bought a big villa in the Algarve in the late sixties and we would always go there every year for our summer holidays. As we all got older, one by one we stopped going and when it was eventually just my mum and dad, they decided not to stay in the villa anymore but instead rented out apartments on the coast about fifteen minutes drive away. They ended up spending about four months of the year out there and got to know hundreds of people and got really good deals on apartment rental prices.
Everyone used to ask them, "Seeing as you like it out there so much, why don't you buy a place?"
My dad would always answer, "What's the point? If we get fed up staying where we are, we can just go somewhere else and we don't have to worry about the upkeep of owning a place"
Anyway, me and mum ended up going and stayed at an apartment my mum and dad had been using for the last couple of years. The housekeeper who worked on the apartments kept a lot of their stuff packed away

and locked up when they weren't there and mum had to sort through it all. It was great to go back there again and I got to meet loads of my mum's friends. They were all really sorry to hear about dad and all said what a nice bloke he was. Mum and dad were really liked out there and had a kind and generous nature about them. If they were driving down a country lane at night in the middle of nowhere and saw someone walking along by the side of the road, they would stop and give them a lift to where they were going. My dad was really good at "weighing people up" and would only stop if he felt the person was okay. They had such a wide range of friends and one of them used to be a Chief Inspector Detective at New Scotland Yard. If anyone knew my dad, they would find that hard to believe but they got on so well and loved telling each other stories about the past. I met him and his wife while we were out there and they were such lovely people. My sister Ellie came out and joined us for about five days and it seemed like going back in time to all those years ago when we'd spend our holidays in Portugal.

March 2010

The woodwork guy did cut down to two days a week and I got paid for the other three (great!)
I was getting more and more back to being my old self but still wasn't fully there yet. Wednesdays are activities day and I would take some of the guys bowling with a volunteer. I'm not really a big fan of the game but it's great to see all these 'proper' bowlers with their own shoes and bowling balls, taking it all seriously and leaving one or two pins up and then one

SECTION 4: GETTING BETTER

of our lot, slinging the ball any old how and it bouncing from side to side off the bumper things like a pin ball machine and getting a strike. You can see these 'pros' looking over at us fuming while we all shout and cheer and holler.

"Get the hosepipe out!" I'll yell when one of the guys gets a strike, "He's on fire!"

I was still having my daughter stay with me and mum for long weekends, once a month and began to notice that it was becoming easier and easier to drive back home on my own once I'd dropped her off to her mum at Fleet. Not that I didn't miss her as much anymore, of course I did and always will but I was becoming more rational and learning how to deal with it. She loves staying with us and we always have a brilliant time because I can fully devote myself to her, doing simple things like going to the New Forest or walking along the sea front.

Peter, the manager at work who gave me the tour the first time I visited the place, is really into the psychological and medical aspects of the service users and we will all often discuss it in the staff room at handover in the mornings and afternoons. I found that I started to become completely fascinated by the whole thing and before I started there, assumed that doctors and experts now knew all there is to know about the brain and human behaviour but so much of it is still a mystery. For instance, we have a girl who comes every day and while she is eating her lunch, will almost every time have petit mals which are a type of seizure. She won't thrash about but sort of switch off and droop her head and hands. A member of staff always sits with her at lunch times and we've tried all different kinds of tactics to try and prevent it from happening but nothing seems to work. She always rushes her food and it's almost as if the eagerness to eat, starts off the petit mals and so we encourage her to take her time and have a drink of water every so often. On occasions, I purposely pretend not to pay much attention and see if by not 'causing a fuss' it makes any difference. The first time I tried it, she didn't have one petit mal and I thought to myself, "That's it, I've cracked it!" but the next time I attempted the same thing, she had about five, one after the other. The doctors just don't know why it's happening and have come up with all these different ideas but nothing seems to work. One of the most common conditions amongst the guys is autism and although I'd heard of it and roughly understood what it meant, didn't really have a clue about how it affected each individual. I've since learnt there are so many different forms and it can take on all manner of characteristics, depending on the individual. I went on this course last year and the Australian lady giving the talk, suffers from autism herself but has still managed to write dozens of books on the subject and gives lectures all over the world. She described how it can affect people and the things they do because most people with the condition, reason in black and white because they hear someone say something and expect it to be exactly how it's said. Her son has autism and when he was younger; his friend (who also has it) came round for tea and they were watching T.V in the living room. When it was ready, she went into the room and said, "Your tea is on the table"

After a couple of minutes, they came into the kitchen and the friend started throwing a tantrum. She asked him what was wrong but he wouldn't answer her and when she asked her son, he said, "He's upset because the food is on a plate and not on the table"

A lot of people with autism take things literally and I could go on for ages about it but I'll leave that to the Australian lady and other people who are much more qualified than I am.

CHAPTER 49

July 2010

The woodwork instructor officially retired at the beginning of the month and a vacancy for the post was put up on the notice board and in the local paper. I immediately applied for it and had my interview the following week, along with about five other people. Although I'd been working there for nearly a year as either a volunteer or part time paid position and knew everyone, I was still really nervous and after the interview, was told that I'd hear something in about a week. I can always remember standing in the kitchen at my mum's house the following week and Dave and Pauline came in. Dave handed me a letter and I nervously opened it and to my sheer delight, it said that I been accepted to the post of new woodwork instructor on a full-time basis. I can't tell you how happy I was. Well......actually that's a lie, I can tell you. I was very happy! I started full time work on Monday, 2nd August 2010 and really felt that I was now part of the team. This was a real boost to my confidence and I think it was at about this point that I was almost back to the old me.

The woodwork and pottery departments were situated in the building facing the courtyard and both rooms were a good size but it was decided that the drama room / dance studio, should now accommodate some of this space, with new toilets and a new reception area being built alongside. There had never really been a drama room before (the dining room was used but this meant constantly putting the tables up and down) and so it made sense. Because of these changes, pottery and woodwork were moved up into the garden buildings which were at that time, used for storage etc. This was fine by me, the only draw back being that the new woodwork room would be considerably smaller but it was going to be fully insulated with central heating and for someone who'd spent most of his working life in freezing cold factories; this was music to my ears. I mean, I wasn't getting any younger and the old bones start to suffer after a while!

One of our first jobs when all the building work had been completed and we'd finally moved in, was to build the stage for the drama / dance studio and all my guys worked really hard on it (I'm so proud of them)

It's in five sections and can be dismantled for when we have our summer fetes and used in the garden. All of the staff are great and we get on really well, helping each other out when needed and I've never worked in a place where everyone is in a good mood nearly all the time. The place has a real relaxed atmosphere to it which is totally intentional because it creates just the right mood and environment for the service users.

September 2010

Every year at the end of August and beginning of September, there is a scarecrow competition held in the village and when you drive through it, you can see everything from Laurel and Hardy (my favourites!) to a queue of people waiting for a bus. The girl in the art department is so talented and she and her guys make our entry to the competition every year, with some help from the lady in craft and her mob. When I first started in 2009, the competition had just started and our scarecrow was Paddington Bear with his suitcase, which made my day because I'm a big fan and read all his books when I was a kid. So now it was time for the competition again and everyone decided that we should have Dastardly and Muttley in their flying machine as our scarecrows. Wow, the art group did a brilliant job! They made the red biplane and stuck it up in a big tree by the drive when you come in and Muttley was falling through the air, with the pigeon flying past him (wearing goggles, a red scarf and carrying the mail bag around his neck)

Dastardly had his legs sticking out the ground, where he'd crashed into the earth and there was a button on the trunk of the tree which when pressed, turned Muttley's tail around like a propeller! We got first prize that year and it was fully deserved because it was up against some strong competition.

About a week later, I got a call from my cousin Lee to say that Roy (a good friend of ours and in particular, Lee's dad Mick) had died and his funeral was in a couple of days' time. Roy's dad had worked for the family business years ago and Roy started when he left school in the sixties. When he got married, he moved to Ireland but eventually came back and worked for us in the nineties. After the funeral, we had a drink in one of Roy's favourite pubs and I told Lee that I was looking to buy a car. He said that he was selling his and so we agreed on a price and after my mum kindly leant me the money, I picked it up on the Saturday. Like I've mentioned before, I'll always be grateful to Dave and for the lifts into work but I

SECTION 4: GETTING BETTER

wanted my independence back again and also, I didn't like to keep asking my mum if I could borrow her car every time I went to pick up my daughter from Fleet. It felt brilliant to have my own wheels again and also because Dave didn't do the handovers at work (he starts before everyone else and so leaves earlier) it became necessary to have my own vehicle so he didn't have to wait for me (not that he would have minded)

My confidence was bouncing back now and when I went to see the psychiatrist, he noticed immediately.

"Do you really need to see me anymore, John?" he asked.

"No, not really but I'll miss our little chats"

"I'm so pleased for you," he said. "everything is working out fine in both your family and work life and always remember, if you ever feel you need to see me, just give me a call"

I stood up and we shook hands and as I headed for the door, I turned around and said, "You know....the first time I met you at my sister's house, I hated your guts"

"I know you did," he replied and laughed.

"Sorry about that"

"Take care John"

"You too mate"

October 2010

It was Halloween again and this time, I wasn't going to let a service user loose with a load of paint on me boat race. The art teacher girl was in her room painting the guy's faces with a friend of hers and I went in and asked if she could put a bullet hole in my forehead.

"Don't tempt me John," she replied.

She started off by slapping a lump of wax on my head and then moulding it into a slight mound with a hole on the middle. Her friend then started to paint it flesh coloured with blood and stuff and it was finished off with a few white splodges, as if the skin around the wound had drained of blood.

When they gave me a mirror to look at the result, I was amazed how realistic it looked. I walked into the tea room at break time and all the guys were asking, "John! John! What's happened to your head?"

"I was walking in the garden and got shot by a sniper"

"Oh no, you must get to hospital straight away!"

"Nah, I'll be all right. It's only a scratch"

"But we can see inside your head!"

"There's not much to see"

"Shall we call an ambulance?"

I couldn't keep a straight face and started laughing, "It's not real, it's make-up for Halloween"

When I got home from work that afternoon, I knocked on the door and Steve answered it. He saw me holding my head and asked, "What's the matter?"

I started groaning and said, "I've just fallen over and hit my head on the door step, could you call an ambulance?" and then removed my hand to reveal the gruesome spectacle.

"Fuck me! Are you all right mate?" he replied.

I started laughing and then he realised it was a joke.

"You bastard!" he mumbled.

It took ages washing it off in the shower and the next day when I went into work, the guys said, "Are you all better now John? Did you go to the hospital?"

"Yes….all better now," I replied.

CHAPTER 50

January 2011

I'd actually had a decent Christmas / New Year, which made a bleedin' change and stayed over with the kids for a couple of nights. It was great to see the boys as they were by now, working long hours and weren't usually around. Early in January, it started to snow quite heavy and because the journey into work comprised of lots of country lanes, quite a few people couldn't make it in. One morning, just as I was leaving home, Dave rang from work and asked if I could pick up a couple of car covers they had on offer at the supermarket near me. When I got there, I found they had a few different types and so rang him back and asked which one's he wanted. I heard my manager call out in the background, "Tell John, no one is coming in today because of the snow. He might as well go home"
"Just a minute," said Dave to my manager, "Why doesn't he go to Arbourfield? You said they needed someone to help out there"
"Oh yes, I'd forgotten about that. Good idea Dave"
Arbourfield is one of three homes owned by the company, situated in Southbourne which have eight residents in each, all with their own bedrooms. There are a further eight bedrooms above the main building where I work and all of these places have their own manager, senior support worker and support workers,

as well as bank staff who cover any shifts when necessary. We also have domiciliary care for people who choose to live independently as well as registered care homes which have 24 hour staff support.

Anyway, just as I thought I could drive back home and put my feet up, Dave says, "Did you hear that John? You can go to Arbourfield and help out there"

"Yeh, I heard. Cheers mate!"

I was only joking and was actually pleased to be going there as I hadn't worked in one of the homes before and thought it would all be good experience. It's quite different supporting the guys in their own home and I really enjoyed it. A couple of days later when the snow had gone and everything was back to normal, I asked the manager of the flats upstairs if I could become a bank support worker and after giving me an interview, he agreed. My thinking was that I'm at work anyway and so when I finish, I don't have to travel anywhere and I could earn some extra money. Most of the shifts I do are in the week from 5pm to 10pm but I occasionally work weekends too. The money isn't brilliant (that's the only downside to the job) but you soon realise money isn't everything and learn to adapt to what you earn. A few weeks later, I was trained to administer the guy's meds and I love my new responsibilities.

April 2011

The lady in charge of organising the timetable for the volunteers asked me if I would like to write a little bit about myself and how I started as a volunteer, before eventually becoming a full member of staff. She said they were updating the website and thought it was a

good idea to find out how people got to know about the place and decided to work there. I agreed, wrote a couple of pages and left it with my manager and thought nothing more about it. He came up to me later in the day and said, "It's really good John but are you sure you want us to use it? It's very personal"
I had to laugh to myself and thought, "Just wait 'til you read the book I'm writing, that's personal"
"Yeh, yeh, that's fine," I answered.
"Thanks John, I think this could inspire others to become volunteers"
I won't show you it all as some of it has already been written here in the book but this is the last part:

My dad passed away at the end of the year and it was then that I realised I should stay with my mum. I eventually got the job as woodwork instructor and can honestly say that I think I've got the best job in the world! Everyone who works for the organisation, either as an employee or a volunteer will tell you the same thing. Working with the service users and getting to know them all as individuals is so rewarding and every day is different. Just say you had a rotten weekend and you wake up Monday morning ready to go to work. It's pouring with rain and freezing cold, so understandably you're not in the best of moods! Within ten minutes of getting to work, you'll be as right as rain!!!!!!

That sums up the whole place really. The guys are just great and if you are feeling a bit low, they know it straight away and soon snap you out of it. Steve had got a job about a mile down the road from my mum's house and had been working there for about six months. He went to a party of one the people he works with and was introduced to his neighbour and eventually started going out with her. She seemed a nice person and Steve was really happy which pleased me because I know he suffers with depression also and has had a bit of a rough time in the past. For the next few months I didn't see him that much as he spent a lot of the time round her house and when I wasn't working overtime, I sat in the kitchen and watched T.V because I had a lot of debts to pay off and couldn't afford to go out very often.

June 2011

I decided that we'd make a 'spectacular' birdhouse for the summer fete coming up at the end of July but didn't know what type of house it should be. One lunch time, I was explaining this to one of the service users and she suggested that it could be a replica of the main building with its distinctive roof and hay loft. I thought it was a brilliant idea and asked if she would like to help, seeing as it was her who thought of it. She agreed and so after lunch, we got working on it straight away. There were only five weeks left until the fete and because I knew it had to be special and the fact that most of the time, I was being asked to do odd jobs around the place, it didn't give us much time. It's become a bit of a joke amongst the staff now that I'm hardly in the woodwork department and I don't really mind doing all of those other jobs because it makes every day different but it's not really fair on the guys in my group. Say I have to put a shelf up in one of the offices, then there are about six blokes following me upstairs, one holding the shelf, one holding a drill, one holding the screw gun (you get the idea) and then you have to try and share out their participations evenly. So one drills the holes, one............(and so on and so forth) The girl who'd suggested the idea of the birdhouse, cut out the shapes of the walls and roof on the band saw, out of plywood and then helped me screw them together. Someone else painted a large piece of card a rusty red colour and then one of the other guys cut out roof tile shapes. By about week three, it was clear the thing wasn't going to get finished in time and so I had to take it home and work on it in the evenings and at weekends. It was completed just in time but it's a real shame that the service user who thought of it, left just before the summer fete and so she never got to see the finished result. I had no idea how much to charge for the birdhouse and so we decided that we'd have an auction and the highest bidder would win it. This unfortunately wasn't a good idea because I felt it was worth at least £100 and so that's what we started the bidding at. Nobody put a bid in, even when we pretended to have an overseas bidder on the phone showing interest and so the guy who was doing the auctioneering, asked me if I'd be prepared to drop the price. I felt that we'd put so much hard work into it and decided not to go below the one hundred.

This year we made a birdhouse resembling the house out of the film "Psycho" and it even has Mrs. Bates at the bedroom window, sitting in a rocking chair which is attached to a pendulum. At the base of the pendulum is a round block of wood with the silhouette of Alfred Hitchcock on it and when it is moved from side to side, Mrs. Bates starts to rock in the chair!

CHAPTER 51

August 2011

At the park in Boscombe they hold a thing every year called Festival of Diversity, which is the only festival to be organised and run by people with learning difficulties. I was asked if I would like to have a woodwork stool there, to show people what we do in our group and thought it would be a good idea to take the birdhouse along. Instead of an auction, I realised the best thing to do was raffle it as people don't mind laying out a couple of quid. In the end, we managed to get £220 but the winning person didn't claim it even after I tried ringing them several times, so it's now in the garden at work and the guys can look at it every day. Result!

The volunteers where I work are amazing and give up so much of their time; it's not as if they've got loads of money or anything. It was a bit different for me because I desperately needed to work to start paying off my debts and so being a volunteer wasn't really a position I could stay in but knew that I didn't want to leave the place. I was doing plenty of overtime at the flats upstairs and was really enjoying it. I even did a few shifts at Pinechurch, which is another one of the houses in Southbourne. On one of the Saturday shifts there, it was the time of the Bournemouth Air Show and me and another member of staff took the guys to the sea front (which is only a 5 minute walk away) to see the display. My shift had started at 2 o'clock and

so we were too late for the Red Arrows but some of the residents of Pinechurch told me that they saw them flying over their garden. I reckon it was probably the hottest day of the year and even when we got to the sea front, there was hardly any breeze. We had a picnic and a lovely time watching all the different planes and helicopters fly past. Steve had told me that morning, he was going to Southbourne as well to watch the display with his girlfriend but I couldn't see him and so gave him a call.
"Where are you boy?" I asked.
"We didn't go in the end," he replied. "Have you seen the news?"
"No, why?"
"One of the Red Arrows has crashed"
"Is the pilot okay?"
"Dunno, they haven't said yet"
After we ended the call, I looked around at all the other people watching the show and could tell that nobody had heard the news yet. I went over to the other member of staff and whispered to her, what I'd been told. All the guys are massive Red Arrow fans and in particular, one of the ladies and I didn't want her to hear anything until I knew more about it. The staff member got the BBC news website up on her phone and confirmed that it was true. By now, lots of the other spectators were talking amongst themselves about the crash and so I decided to tell the guys. The female service user who absolutely loves the Red Arrows became quite upset and so I tried to reassure her by saying that they didn't know about the pilot yet and said that, "no news is good news"
When we got back to the house, she kept asking me to look on the news website but every time I did, there

was no mention of how the pilot was. This went on for about three hours but after tea and meds, she went up to her room and had a lay down. I checked the BBC news website about an hour later and it said that the pilot had been killed. While I was reading this, one of the other service users looked over my shoulder and read it too.

"Don't say anything to you know who," I told her, "let her sleep and she'll find out about it in the morning"

I must admit that she was good and didn't go and tell her but made sure that the rest of the guys found out.

"Guess what, guess what!" she yelled, "The pilot was killed!"

"Keep your voice down," I said, "you'll wake her up"

My shift finished a short while later and when I got home, I sat in the kitchen and had a few beers. Steve came in at just after midnight and said that he'd been to a party and had a massive argument with his girlfriend. I told him that it would all blow over but he said they'd been arguing a lot lately and were definitely finished. On the Monday at work, all the guys were really upset about the pilot's death and so the lady who runs the craft department, made a plaque and they held a short service in the sensory garden. Apart from the sad feeling amongst the service users and staff, I was feeling really good in myself (the first time in as long as I could remember) and now felt that my confidence was back 100%. Because of the split with his girlfriend, Steve was back at home again and he was really miserable. He was obviously still very fond of her but said that she didn't want him back. On the Thursday evening I was working upstairs at the flats and making myself a cup of coffee in the kitchen,

SECTION 4: GETTING BETTER

when my phone rang. I didn't recognise the number and when I answered it and the person said, "Is that John?" I didn't recognise the voice either.
"Yeh"
"This is Steve's ex girlfriend"
"Hello"
"Sorry to bother you because you're probably at work"
"Yeh, I am. What's wrong?"
"You know Steve a lot better than I do and I've just received a phone call from him"
"Oh right"
"He's threatened to kill himself"
"Oh"
"The thing is, I don't know if he means it or is it just an attempt to try and get back with me?"
"I really don't know but I think he's attempted it in the past. Don't worry, I'll ring his mum and let her know"
"Thanks John, sorry to bother you at work"
"No worries"
Luckily, all the residents were either in their bedrooms or watching T.V in the lounge and the other staff member was sorting out meds. I went into the office and phoned my sister's number and it was answered by Dave. I relayed the info and then told him that I had to go because I was supposed to be working. For the rest of my shift, I couldn't stop thinking about Steve and hoped he was okay. I knew what it was like to be really low and he'd often told me about his depression.

CHAPTER 52

When I got home, I walked into the kitchen and Steve was sitting at the dining table drinking a can of Super Tennants and listening to the radio on the T.V. He didn't look up at me and I didn't really know what to say to him and so I made my mum a cup of tea and took it into the living room, where she was watching television. I then went back into the kitchen, got myself a beer from the fridge and went outside to the garden for a cigarette. When I'd finished smoking, I went back in, pulled out a chair and sat opposite him.
"All right?" I asked.
I won't go into the details but let's just say that he really started to have a go at me and I thought to myself, "For fucks sake! It's twenty past ten at night, I've just got in from work and now I'm getting all this abuse!"
I really had no idea why he had it in for me and went into the living room and said to my mum, "He's going mad at me in there and I don't need it. Ring his mum up and tell her to get round here, let her deal with it"
It was Thursday night and I'd taken the Friday off as holiday because my daughter was coming for the weekend and the Monday was a bank holiday, so that meant I could have her for four days but there was no way now that I could let her come and stay. I walked into the hallway and rang my wife's number. Steve came out of the kitchen and said, "Who the fuck are you ringing?"

SECTION 4: GETTING BETTER

"My daughter. She was supposed to be staying this weekend but now I'm going to have to cancel it"

I won't tell you what he said next but after I'd spoke to my wife and gave some excuse about having to work over the weekend, I went back into the living room. While my mum was ringing Pauline, Steve came in and continued having a go at me.

"Oi, Oi Steve….language! I'm trying to watch Eastenders here," said my mum who calmly sat there and continued watching the T.V.

Steve was saying something along the lines of, "Come outside, come outside. What…are you afraid of me?"

For the first time in ages, I'd got my life sorted out and had a job I absolutely loved. There was no way I was going to risk all of that by having a fight with some drunk bloke. Who knows what would have happened, we could have ended up getting nicked and I would have lost my job for sure. That thought terrified me because I knew I would never get a job like that again. Steve had his nose almost touching mine and was swearing his head off but I kept as calm as I could and said, "Why are you speaking to me like this, what have I done to you?"

A couple of minutes later, Pauline and Dave walked into the room and she told Steve to go into the kitchen with her. I stayed in the living room for about another ten minutes but was desperate for a fag and another beer and so went into the kitchen where Pauline and Steve were sitting at the table, walked past them, got a beer and went into the garden. All of a sudden I became aware that my legs were starting to shake and then the whole of my body. I had to really concentrate and clench my teeth and fists together, to try and stop it happening. My mind started racing at 100mph because I was so angry and was repeatedly telling myself, "Calm down John, fucking calm down!"

Steve came outside with his mum behind him and I honestly thought he was going to apologise to me but instead, he continued swearing and saying, "Come on then, come on then!"

He'd obviously had a lot to drink but I was completely sober and was 100% ready for him to come at me. All I was going to do was quickly move to one side, trip him up and then……….

That's the bit that really got me scared because I was ready to really hurt him badly when he was on the floor. Forget all that stuff about who's harder than who, I can't stand that rubbish. It's the sort of thing that teenagers say and I'm definitely not much cop at fighting. Trip him up, let him fall on the patio floor and kick him hard in the head, over and over and over again! That was my plan.

As he swore at me, Pauline told him to go back inside, which fortunately he did and as he made his way into the kitchen, she said, "I'm so sorry John"

"You've got nothing to apologise about, it's not your fault," I replied.

Pauline went back indoors and I stayed in the garden, smoking one cigarette after the other, trying to calm down and saying to myself, "Don't react John, don't be a prick! I mustn't fuck everything up and lose my job! I can't lose my job, I can't lose my job, I mustn't lose my job!"

Steve came back out into the garden about fifteen minutes later and said, "Sorry John, I'm being a total wanker. I've got nothing against you, I fucking love you!"

"Don't worry about it," I replied but inside I was thinking, "I ain't fucking trusting you any more mate!"

We went back into the kitchen, sat at the table and both opened a can of beer each. I was drinking normal stuff while Steve was still on the Super T's and he seemed much more subdued. We talked for about thirty minutes and then I told him that I had to go to the toilet and on the way back, I popped my head around the living room door and told Pauline that he was much calmer now and they could go home. Back in the kitchen, me and Steve carried on drinking but I made sure I was only sipping mine and when he was ready for another, I told him I'd get it from the fridge. While I was there, I poured the rest of mine down the sink and then got us both another one each, pretending that I'd finished mine the same time as his. That man sure can drink because he finished all his beers and then started on mine and I thought, "Ain't he ever gonna go to fuckin' bed?"

I can't remember what we were talking about (a load of crap probably) and I kept staring at his face, looking for signs of tiredness. By about 2am, his eyes were beginning to droop and I noticed he'd stopped drinking but instead, had his head down, staring at the kitchen floor. I took his glass away, went to the fridge and topped it up again.

"Here you are boy, have another one," I said as I put the glass down in front of him.

He was almost asleep by now but still managed to lift the glass to his mouth and take a couple of gulps. I wanted to sleep soundly in the knowledge that the rest of the night would be uneventful and was determined to get him unconscious. At about half two I went into the garden for a smoke and watched him through the kitchen window. His chin was now on his chest and his arms were drooped by his side but I noticed his leg was shaking and knew he was still full of rage. At 3am he finally fell asleep at the kitchen table and I called out loudly, "Steve, go to bed!"

He slowly lifted his head and replied, "Yeh, I'm knackered," and then went upstairs.

I sat at the kitchen table until I could hear him snoring and then stayed up for another couple of hours because I was still sober and needed a good drink myself!

The next morning, I woke up at 8am and realised Steve was still asleep and so went into his bedroom and woke him up, telling him he was late for work.

"Oh shit!" he replied.

I went downstairs and made myself a cup of tea and a little while later, Steve came down and said, "Could you give me a lift to work, I'm really late"

"I can't Steve," I answered, "I've only had a couple of hours sleep and I'm still over the limit"

"But I'll get the sack if I'm late again"

"What about me? I'll get the sack if I'm done for drink driving"

"For fucks sake!" he shouted, "You don't care about me!"

"Come on then, let's go"

I just wanted him out of the house and didn't want to get into an argument. We got in the car and I drove him to work and all the way, we hardly said a word. When we pulled up outside, he got out and said, "Thanks mate, I'll see you later"

"No you won't," I thought to myself and drove back home.

SECTION 5: BETTER?

CHAPTER 53

I was extremely pissed off about not being to able to see my daughter and was really angry the way Steve had talked to me and threatened me. When I got back home, my mum was up and I told her that I'd taken Steve to work.
"What's up with him?" she asked.
"Dunno"
Now I didn't have to pick up my daughter from Fleet and I wasn't working, I was at a loose end and this left me too much time on my hands and so I couldn't stop thinking about the previous evening. As the day went on, I found I was getting more and more agitated with the thought of seeing Steve when he got in from work. I didn't want to hear his apologies (not that he would have probably given any) and was so annoyed with him, I just couldn't face seeing him. I phoned my wife and explained the real reason I'd cancelled my daughter's visit and she agreed I'd made the right decision. It got to about 4:15 in the afternoon and he was due home in half an hour. My whole body started shaking again and I was beginning to really panic and so I went to my mum and told her that I had to go.
"Why?"
"I can't face seeing him"
"You could stay round Pauline's and I'll tell him that he has to move out tomorrow"
"That's no good, he's bound to go round there tonight and say sorry to her"
"Where are you gonna go then?"

SECTION 5: BETTER?

"I'll give Ellie a ring and go round there. I doubt if he'll guess I'm staying at her place and it's not that easy getting a train or bus to Southbourne"

"Don't worry John, there's no way he's staying here, not after last night. You're my son anyway, you come first"

"Thanks mum"

So I rang my sister Ellie and she said it was okay for me to stay. I got an overnight bag, packed a load of beers and fags (and a few clothes) put the laptop in the car and reversed out of the drive. In my rear-view mirror, I could see Steve walking up the road and quickly drove away. As soon as I turned the corner and knew I wouldn't be seeing him face to face, I immediately started to calm down but still wasn't right. On the way to Ellie's house, I pulled into the surgery car park where Pauline works and asked the receptionist if I could see her quickly. When Pauline came down, I told her how anxious I was feeling and was it possible for me to see my doctor straight away.

"I'll see what I can do John," she said, "Wait here and I'll ask him as soon as his next patient comes out"

"Cheers Paul"

When the doctor was free, Pauline came up to me and whispered that I could go in. He's a really nice bloke and was very understanding when I gave him the gist of what had happened and how I was feeling. He prescribed me 5mg tablets of Olanzapine which is an antipsychotic and lessens the feelings of anxiousness. It is also used to treat all the symptoms associated with bipolar disorder and was in fact, the drug I was first prescribed before changing over to Sodium Valproate. When I'd been taking the Olanzapine every day, I felt that it was causing me to put on a lot of weight. I spoke to my psychiatrist about this and he said weight gain can be one of the side effects and so that's why I made the switch. In hindsight I don't think the weight gain was anything to do with the tablets but instead due to the fact I wasn't working, lack of exercise and stuffing myself stupid on a regular basis! When I got to Ellie's I told her everything that had happened with Steve and could feel myself getting all worked up again. I'd forgotten to take an Olanzapine tablet and so swallowed one straight away. Within half an hour I felt completely calm again and guessed that taking that, along with the Sodium Valproate I was using every night, must have doubled the effectiveness and speed of recovery. Anyway, who cares…….it worked! I crashed out on Ellie's sofa that night and in the morning, felt fine and didn't feel the need to take another tablet. I was still really angry with Steve because I was sure he didn't realise what he'd done to me. All that time it took to get me back on an even keel and in the space of ten minutes, I was right back to how I felt when I was discharged from the hospital. I'm sure Steve didn't really mean all of those things and although I was cross with him, I still love the big brute (I must be bleedin' bonkers!)

Before that Thursday evening, I was only taking one tablet per night of the Sodium Valproate but now I was back on the anti-depressants as well as the Olanzapine. I'd really felt that I was back to my old self and if anything, even better than my old self but now I was a nervous fucking wreck! My mum rang me at Ellie's and said that Steve had gone out for the day, arranging for a place to go and live and would be moving out the following day. So I spent the night at my sister's again and we had a game where I played

SECTION 5: BETTER?

loads of obscure theme tunes on my laptop and she had to guess which films they were from. She wasn't very good at it but I must admit that I'm a bit of a sad old git when it comes to do with anything about films. The next morning, I drove back to my mum's house and was sitting in the kitchen, when Steve came in the front door. He went straight upstairs and started putting all his belongings on the front doorstep. This took him about twenty minutes and when he'd finished and closed the front door behind him, he sent me a text saying, "I NEVER WANT 2 SPEAK 2 U AGAIN, U BIG BABY!"

I had a spare sim card in the drawer and immediately changed it over with my usual one. If he didn't want to speak to me then fine; I wasn't that keen on speaking to him either.

Monday was the August bank holiday and now Steve had left, I was feeling fine and so didn't bother taking any of the Olanzapine. At work on Tuesday and everyone seemed so loud and 'in your face' although most of the staff say the same thing when they've been off for a few days. I suppose it's like that all the time but you just get used to it and usually after a couple of hours, it all seems normal again. Lunchtime can usually be pretty noisy but on this occasion, to me it was deafening. We all sat in the dining room (staff and service users alike) and there were six people to a table. I was sitting next to another member of staff and all I seemed to be hearing from the guys was, "John, what do you think of this?" or, "John, what are we doing this afternoon?" etc.

It really got to me and I think I was starting to get what I can only describe as another panic attack. I've not had them that often (only really once before in my flat or possibly twice, when I met Pauline and my mum in Subways) and had to put my knife and fork down because I was shaking. The other staff member asked if I was okay but I didn't answer and immediately got up and went into the kitchen. People seemed to be milling about everywhere and I couldn't stand the noise. Luckily I saw Peter (my day service manager) talking to Dave and I noticed that Dave had left his office door open, which was just besides the kitchen. I got Peter's attention and motioned my arm for him to come into the office. He asked me if everything was okay and I explained that I had to go home (he knew about my bipolar) so I could take an Olanzapine. Peter completely understood and told me to take the rest of the day off, "Just make sure you bring the tablets into work with you tomorrow," he said.

So that's exactly what I did and took them probably for about the next fortnight. I really didn't want to take them for any longer than I had to and slowly weaned myself off them until I felt I was back to normal again. Peter is such a great bloke and we often have discussions about bipolar, which he says is, "Just a chemical imbalance in the brain"

Some of the service users have it but because of their learning difficulties, they don't really understand why they are suffering from the symptoms. Peter had once said to me, "I think I've got Bipolar Lite!"

"What do you mean?" I'd asked.

"Because when I go out on a Friday night and walk into a wine bar, I shout out 'champagne for everyone!"

"Yep….that sounds about right"

CHAPTER 54

August 2012

Nearly a year has passed since that incident with Steve. I'm feeling really good in myself and am still doing quite a lot of shift work in the upstairs flats. I went to see my daughter a few weeks ago on her birthday and both my boys were there too. We had a really great time and later on in the evening, they had some mates round for a drink and I couldn't help noticing what nice people they were. They all get on really well with my daughter and said, "HAPPY BIRTHDAY NIN!" (Our nickname for her) and were so polite and friendly. My wife has done a great job with the kids since I've left and we get on really well too. We're good mates now and that's the best way to be if possible.

I'm so proud to be a part of the team where I work and would like to thank the guys in particular, for making me a better person. They will never know how they've altered my outlook on life and I love their honesty and kindness. Of course, some of them can be hard work and be spiteful and deceitful sometimes (just like anybody else) but for the most part, they are just great! I've changed; I'm not the same person I used to be. The side of me that's always messing about and not taking things too seriously is still there but something has gone and I'm really pleased about it. About two months ago I bought the film "Tyrannosaur" directed by Paddy Considine and the acting (Olivia Colman in particular) is outstanding. I won't go into the story line much but her character has an abusive husband and in one scene, he hits her and then rapes her in their bedroom. Of course, this is shocking enough but I actually found the scene where he arrives home late, much more powerful. We see her character a couple of hours earlier, sitting on the sofa drinking a glass of wine and then it cuts to him opening the front door. He is drunk and loudly calling out her name, then goes to the living room and keeps switching the light on and off, still calling her name in a piss taking tone. The camera then cuts to her sleeping on the sofa with the wine bottle standing on the coffee table, nearly empty. It's a low camera angle and we see him stand in front of her and urinate all over her fully clothed body. He walks away and out of shot but the camera is still on Olivia Colman's character. When we hear but can't see he has left the room, she opens her eyes and just lies there. To me that scene reveals all about their relationship without having to show him abusing and raping her. She would rather pretend to be asleep and not confront him, which tells us what a total cunt he must be. If I had seen that film a few months earlier, then my reaction would have been, "I want to kill the fucker!" but instead, after watching it I felt sadness instead of anger. I wanted to know why he'd become that way toward her and wished that his family really knew what he was like. Of course, he made me feel sick but the thought of actually killing him, made me feel even worse. That's the part of me that has changed. I would once have wanted to hurt him badly but that feeling has completely vanished. I don't like violence (never have) but felt it was acceptable to punish someone with violence when they had done

SECTION 5: BETTER?

such a terrible thing. Not any more.

It's now possible with the internet, to see images and videos of people in all manner of horrible deaths. Why would anyone want to look at that, it doesn't make any sense? I want that character in the film punished by sending him to prison for life with no chance of parole. I'm definitely not saying that my feelings are the right and only way; everyone is different. If a parent of a child who's been murdered, wants revenge by killing the perpetrator, then who am I to argue? I can fully appreciate why they'd feel that way and wouldn't do anything to try and talk them out of it. I'm just pleased that I have somehow found a sort of inner peace and find it funny that Lucy and Stewart from the hospital and all their attempts at trying to turn me to religion, needn't have bothered. I don't need religion. John Lennon had it figured; just listen to the words of 'Imagine'

Bipolar disorder is relatively easy to live with if you remember to take the medication, even though it did take me ages to appreciate that. I suppose I'm lucky I didn't discover I had bipolar until I got to forty; it must be so hard for someone in their teens or early twenties. All they want to do is go out and have a good time and it's only natural that they forget or don't want to take their meds. Like I've just said, it took a long time for me to be convinced because I totally refused to accept I had a mental illness but now I just don't care and I'm not bothered what anybody else thinks either.

So if a fellow sufferer asked me what my advice would be?

Two things really. The first is to except you have the condition but equally as important, take your medication; I really can't stress that enough. I know when being initially diagnosed, there are many of you who won't agree with that judgement but you have to trust the doctors and psychiatrists….after all, they are there to help you. By all means question it but listen carefully to what they have to say. Of course there is the possibility they might be wrong but still agree to take the tablets nonetheless. Doing so won't kill you and if you do then start to feel better, then you know you're doing the right thing. Good luck.

Anyway, that's my little story.

I hope you enjoyed it.

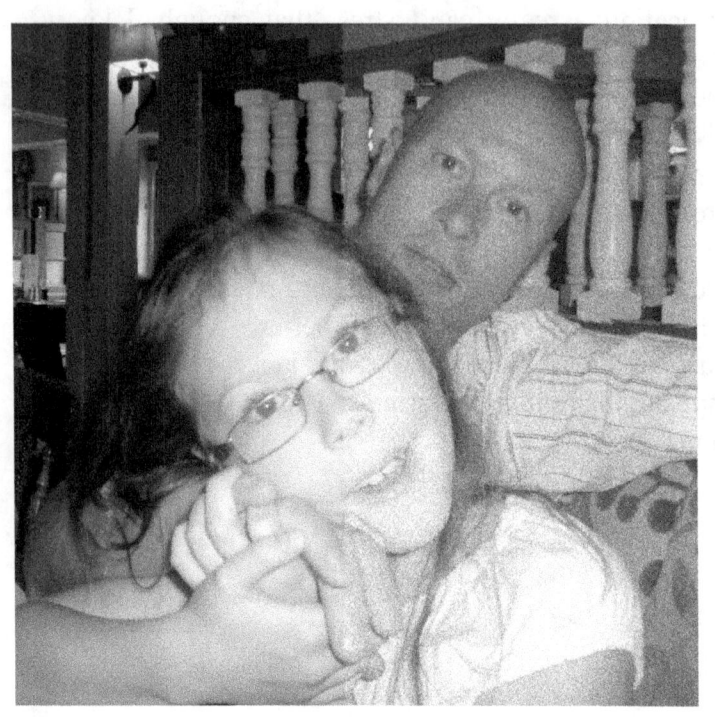

Me and Nin 2012

www.ingramcontent.com/pod-product-compliance
Lightning Source LLC
Chambersburg PA
CBHW061502180526
45171CB00001B/7